MENTORING OF BLACK GRADUATE AND MEDICAL STUDENTS, POSTDOCTORAL SCHOLARS, AND EARLY-CAREER FACULTY IN SCIENCE, ENGINEERING, AND MEDICINE

PROCEEDINGS OF A WORKSHOP

Randall C. Morgan, Jr., Joan Y. Reede, and Paula Whitacre,
Rapporteurs

Cato T. Laurencin, *Editor*

Roundtable on Black Men and Black Women in
Science, Engineering, and Medicine

Policy and Global Affairs

Health and Medicine Division

The National Academies of
SCIENCES • ENGINEERING • MEDICINE

THE NATIONAL ACADEMIES PRESS
Washington, DC
www.nap.edu

THE NATIONAL ACADEMIES PRESS 500 Fifth Street, NW Washington, DC 20001

This activity was supported by contracts between the National Academy of Sciences and Aetna Foundation (#18-8876), Johnson & Johnson, the National Institutes of Health (HHSN263201800029I/75N98021F00006), the National Research Council President's Circle Fund, the University of Pittsburgh, and the W. K. Kellogg Foundation. Any opinions, findings, conclusions, or recommendations expressed in this publication do not necessarily reflect the views of any organization or agency that provided support for the project.

International Standard Book Number-13: 978-0-309-27713-6
International Standard Book Number-10: 0-309-27713-2
Digital Object Identifier: https://doi.org/10.17226/26462

Additional copies of this publication are available from the National Academies Press, 500 Fifth Street, NW, Keck 360, Washington, DC 20001; (800) 624-6242 or (202) 334-3313; http://www.nap.edu.

Printed in the United States of America

Suggested citation: National Academies of Sciences, Engineering, and Medicine. 2022. *Mentoring of Black Graduate and Medical Students, Postdoctoral Scholars, and Early-Career Faculty in Science, Engineering, and Medicine: Proceedings of a Workshop.* Washington, DC: The National Academies Press. https://doi.org/10.17226/26462.

The National Academies of

SCIENCES • ENGINEERING • MEDICINE

The **National Academy of Sciences** was established in 1863 by an Act of Congress, signed by President Lincoln, as a private, nongovernmental institution to advise the nation on issues related to science and technology. Members are elected by their peers for outstanding contributions to research. Dr. Marcia McNutt is president.

The **National Academy of Engineering** was established in 1964 under the charter of the National Academy of Sciences to bring the practices of engineering to advising the nation. Members are elected by their peers for extraordinary contributions to engineering. Dr. John L. Anderson is president.

The **National Academy of Medicine** (formerly the Institute of Medicine) was established in 1970 under the charter of the National Academy of Sciences to advise the nation on medical and health issues. Members are elected by their peers for distinguished contributions to medicine and health. Dr. Victor J. Dzau is president.

The three Academies work together as the **National Academies of Sciences, Engineering, and Medicine** to provide independent, objective analysis and advice to the nation and conduct other activities to solve complex problems and inform public policy decisions. The National Academies also encourage education and research, recognize outstanding contributions to knowledge, and increase public understanding in matters of science, engineering, and medicine.

Learn more about the National Academies of Sciences, Engineering, and Medicine at **www.nationalacademies.org**.

The National Academies of
SCIENCES • ENGINEERING • MEDICINE

Consensus Study Reports published by the National Academies of Sciences, Engineering, and Medicine document the evidence-based consensus on the study's statement of task by an authoring committee of experts. Reports typically include findings, conclusions, and recommendations based on information gathered by the committee and the committee's deliberations. Each report has been subjected to a rigorous and independent peer-review process and it represents the position of the National Academies on the statement of task.

Proceedings published by the National Academies of Sciences, Engineering, and Medicine chronicle the presentations and discussions at a workshop, symposium, or other event convened by the National Academies. The statements and opinions contained in proceedings are those of the participants and are not endorsed by other participants, the planning committee, or the National Academies.

For information about other products and activities of the National Academies, please visit www.nationalacademies.org/about/whatwedo.

MENTORING AND ADVISING ACTION GROUP PLANNING COMMITTEE

RANDALL C. MORGAN, JR. (*Co-chair*), W. Montague Cobb/NMA Health Institute
JOAN Y. REEDE (NAM) (*Co-chair*), Harvard Medical School
MONICA HALL, Robert Wood Johnson Foundation
MaCALUS V. HOGAN, University of Pittsburgh Medical Center
LYNNE M. HOLDEN, Montefiore Medical Center
ORLANDO KIRTON, Abington Jefferson Health
VALERAE LEWIS, University of Texas MD Anderson Cancer Center
WENDY L. YALLOWITZ, Robert Wood Johnson Foundation

Project Staff

REGINALD HAYES, Associate Program Officer, Roundtable on Black Men and Black Women in Science, Engineering, and Medicine
TOM ARRISON, Program Director, Policy and Global Affairs (until May 2021)
PAULA W. WHITACRE, Consultant Writer

ROUNDTABLE ON BLACK MEN AND BLACK WOMEN IN SCIENCE, ENGINEERING, AND MEDICINE

CATO T. LAURENCIN (NAS/NAE/NAM) (*Chair*), University of Connecticut Health
OLUJIMI AJIJOLA, UCLA Medical Center
GILDA A. BARABINO (NAE/NAM), Olin College of Engineering
CHARLES R. BRIDGES, JR., Janssen Research & Development, LLC
CEDRIC BRIGHT, East Carolina University
L. D. BRITT (NAM), Eastern Virginia Medical School
ANDRÉ L. CHURCHWELL, Vanderbilt University School of Medicine
THEODORE CORBIN, Drexel University
GEORGE Q. DALEY (NAM), Harvard Medical School
WAYNE FREDERICK, Howard University
PAULA T. HAMMOND (NAS/NAE/NAM), Massachusetts Institute of Technology
EVELYNN M. HAMMONDS (NAM), Harvard University
LYNNE M. HOLDEN, Montefiore Medical Center
CAMARA P. JONES, Morehouse School of Medicine
CORA BAGLEY MARRETT, University of Wisconsin–Madison
VALERIE MONTGOMERY RICE (NAM), Morehouse School of Medicine
RANDALL C. MORGAN, JR., W. Montague Cobb/NMA Health Institute
ELIZABETH O. OFILI (NAM), Morehouse School of Medicine
VIVIAN W. PINN (NAM), National Institutes of Health (Retired)
JOAN Y. REEDE (NAM), Harvard Medical School
LOUIS W. SULLIVAN (NAM), Morehouse School of Medicine
HANNAH VALANTINE (NAM), Stanford University
CLYDE W. YANCY (NAM), Northwestern University
MARK ALEXANDER (Ex Officio Member), 100 Black Men of America, Inc.
MARIE BERNARD (Ex Officio Member), National Institutes of Health
KIMBERLY BRYANT (Ex Officio Member), Black Girls CODE
IVORY DEAN (Ex Officio Member), Chan Zuckerberg Initiative
GARTH N. GRAHAM (NAM) (Ex Officio Member), Google, Inc.
IAN HENRY (Ex Officio Member), Procter & Gamble Company

Preface

It is an honor for me to serve as chair of the National Academies of Sciences, Engineering, and Medicine Roundtable on Black Men and Black Women in Science, Engineering, and Medicine, and serve as the editor of the second in a series of proceedings publications from the Roundtable. Our work in this space began in 2015 when I and leaders of the W. Montague Cobb/National Medical Association Health Institute recognized the growing absence of Black men in medical schools. In fact, levels of Black men entering medical school reached a historic low in 2015 and 2016. Starting in 2016, and with financial support from important partners such as the Aetna Foundation, the Burroughs Wellcome Fund, the Robert Wood Johnson Foundation, and the Connecticut Legislative Black and Puerto Rican Caucus, we began planning a National Academies workshop on issues surrounding the absence of Black men in medicine. The joint workshop titled "The Growing Absence of Black Men in Medicine and Science" took place in 2017. It was historic, in that to my knowledge, it was the first National Academies activity specifically focused on issues involving Black people. The proceedings volume was titled *An American Crisis: The Growing Absence of Black Men in Medicine and Science*. It was released in May 2018 and corresponded with a briefing on the subject of Black men and medicine with the Congressional Black Caucus in Washington, D.C. Many of the ideas that emerged from the workshop have been embraced by academia, industry, and philanthropy. More needs to be done.

Our next steps have involved the development of a more permanent presence in the National Academies to discuss issues surrounding Black Men and Black Women in Science, Engineering, and Medicine. With support from our anchor partners named above, along with the Johnson & Johnson Company, the W. K. Kellogg Foundation, and the University of Pittsburgh, and with continued leadership and commitment from Dr. Victor J. Dzau, President of the National Academy of Medicine, the Roundtable on Black Men and Black Women in Science, Engineering, and Medicine was launched late in 2018. I am grateful to the steering committee members for the Roundtable: Drs. L. D. Britt, Cedric M. Bright, George Q. Daley, Randall C. Morgan Jr., Elizabeth O. Ofili, Vivian W. Pinn, and Louis W. Sullivan.

In December 2020, the Roundtable organized a workshop aimed at exploring current models used for mentoring and advising. A critical analysis of the effectiveness of mentoring techniques and models took place. Discussions focused on examining the effects of structural barriers such as systemic racism in achieving goals.

I am grateful to the co-chairs of the workshop, Dr. Randall C. Morgan Jr. and Dr. Joan Y. Reede. They worked hard to put in place successfully an innovative workshop and create new ideas and new information on mentoring and advising. I am particularly impressed by their work to bring institutional leadership to bear on issues of successful mentoring. The workshop also embraced "science, engineering, and medicine" to the fullest extent. Participants discussed ideas from pipeline programs to career advising and development from the standpoint of broad areas involving the academic and scientific enterprise. Their discussions present new information and ideas on concepts of advising, mentorship, and sponsorship, while breaking new ground through important mentor-mentee conversations that are featured in these proceedings.

Cato T. Laurencin, M.D., Ph.D. (NAS/NAE/NAM)
Chair, Roundtable on Black Men and Black Women
in Science, Engineering, and Medicine
University Professor, University of Connecticut

Acknowledgments

This Proceedings of a Workshop was prepared by the workshop rapporteurs as a factual summary of what was presented and discussed at the workshop. The planning committee's role was limited to planning and convening the workshop. The statements made are those of the rapporteurs and do not necessarily represent positions of the workshop participants as a whole, the planning committee, or the National Academies of Sciences, Engineering, and Medicine. We wish to extend sincere thanks to all the members of the planning committee for their contributions in scoping, developing, and carrying out this project.

This proceedings has been reviewed in draft form by individuals chosen for their diverse perspectives and technical expertise, in accordance with procedures approved by the National Academies of Sciences, Engineering, and Medicine's Report Review Committee. The purpose of this independent review is to provide candid and critical comments to assist the institution in making its published report as sound as possible and ensure the document meets institutional standards for quality and objectivity. The review comments and draft manuscript remain confidential to protect the integrity of the process. We wish to thank the following individuals for their review of this proceedings: Juan E. Gilbert, University of Florida; Melissa McDaniels, University of Wisconsin–Madison; and Darla Thompson, American Association for the Advancement of Science. Although the reviewers listed above have provided many constructive comments and suggestions, they were not asked to endorse the content of the proceedings, nor did they see the final draft before its release. The review of this proceedings was overseen by Maxine Hayes, University of Washington. Appointed by the National Academies, she was responsible for making certain that an independent examination of this report was carried out in accordance with institutional procedures and that all review comments were carefully considered. Responsibility for the final content of this proceedings rests entirely with the rapporteurs and the institution.

Contents

1

Introduction

Many participants in the workshops and other events held by the Roundtable on Black Men and Black Women in Science, Engineering, and Medicine of the National Academies of Sciences, Engineering, and Medicine have credited relationships with mentors as important to their academic and career development. In further recognition of the importance of mentorship, most, if not all, of these individuals themselves serve as mentors to those who are following in their paths. In addition, many workshop presenters have described mentorship and advising as components of their organizations' broader pathway programs to increase the numbers of Black and other underrepresented minorities in the fields of science, engineering, and medicine.

As described in a recent consensus report from the National Academies on the science of mentoring, "mentorship refers to a collaborative learning relationship and working alliance based on intentionality, trust, and shared responsibility of the interactions in that relationship and the effectiveness of those interactions" (NASEM, 2019, 4), while "advising typically provides feedback about specific questions" (NASEM, 2019, 38). In fulfilling its mission to identify barriers and opportunities encountered by Black men and Black women in entering and succeeding in science, engineering, and medicine careers, the Roundtable recognizes mentoring and advising as promising practices that would benefit from a closer focus. One of its six action groups is dedicated to the topic.

On December 7 and 8, 2020, this action group of the Roundtable took the lead to convene a virtual workshop that examined how to strengthen mentoring and advising of Black students and professionals in science, engineering, and medicine (see Box 1-1 for the Statement of Task). Presenters included faculty deans, social scientists who are experts in organizational and professional development, and program implementers. Throughout the workshop, individual presenters highlighted evaluation criteria used by successful pipeline programs, including statistics on recruitment, retention, and advancement; career and leadership accomplishments; and awards and publications. Breakout groups and a series of three mentor-mentee conversations amplified the points expressed during the presentations and discussions. (See Appendix A for the agenda.)

OPENING REMARKS

Cato T. Laurencin, M.D., Ph.D., University of Connecticut and chair of the Roundtable, welcomed the participants to the workshop and introduced John L. Anderson, Ph.D., National Academy of Engineering (NAE), to open the workshop.

As president of the NAE, Dr. Anderson noted that the National Academies have become more proactive in discussion of and action on issues related to diversity, equity, and inclusion. One example is an NAE committee formed around racial justice and equity in engineering. He noted its creation was driven by NAE members to seek actionable recommendations

BOX 1-1
Statement of Task

Participants will explore the current models used for mentoring and advising (with well-articulated outcomes), and the effectiveness of those models, with a particular focus on the reality of structural barriers and systemic racism.

Discussions will also address the role of institutional leadership in the academic setting in strengthening mentoring and advising. Major objectives of the workshop will include (1) to examine the criteria needed to evaluate a successful pipeline program for Black people pursuing education and careers in science, engineering, and medicine; and (2) to explore the definitions and practices of mentoring, advising, sponsorship, and related roles in order to clarify their functions.

not only for the NAE but also in the broader engineering community. He said he and others in the leadership of the National Academies are looking to the Roundtable on Black Men and Black Women in Science, Engineering, and Medicine for input.

Turning to the topic of the current workshop, Dr. Anderson said he has often served as a mentor or advisor throughout his career. He stressed mentoring is a critical component of career growth, and its importance does not end at graduation, as the workshop agenda recognizes. Considering the origin of the term from Greek mythology (Mentor helped guide the son of Odysseus when the latter went off to fight the Trojan War), Dr. Anderson said, "Mentoring is about building confidence, developing self-esteem, and navigating life. It continues throughout life as mentor or mentee." From the perspective of a white male, he added, he realizes he has had unfair advantages, which he considers when mentoring individuals from other racial backgrounds.

Dr. Laurencin thanked Dr. Anderson, colleagues on the Roundtable, National Academies staff, and the more than 500 participants who registered for the workshop. He reviewed the Roundtable's origins and previous work. The Roundtable grew out of a workshop hosted by the National Academies on the absence of Black men in medicine. In 2016–2017, only 273 African American men were enrolled in medical school, out of more than 21,000 students, according to data compiled by the Association of American Medical Colleges. This led to a workshop and influential report *An American Crisis: The Growing Absence of Black Men in Medicine and Science: Proceedings of a Joint Workshop* (NASEM, 2018b). After release of the report, Dr. Laurencin explained, the Roundtable was launched in 2019 to understand the broader issues impacting Black men and Black women in science, engineering, and medicine, and to create ideas for solutions utilizing the strengths in having Black men and Black women in these fields.

The members of the Roundtable established action groups to share information, engage with key stakeholders, and conduct workshops and other activities for meaningful change. In addition to the mentorship and advising, the other action groups address public engagement, systematic change to avoid psychological barriers, racism and bias, pre-K to graduate education, financing, and, as a later addition, the COVID-19 pandemic.[1]

---

[1] For the Roundtable's activities and previous reports, see https://www.nationalacademies.org/our-work/roundtable-on-black-men-and-black-women-in-science-engineering-and-medicine.

FRAMING COMMENTS FROM THE WORKSHOP CO-CHAIRS

Workshop co-chair Randall C. Morgan, Jr., M.D., M.B.A., Cobb/NMA Health Institute, welcomed participants. He noted that developing the workshop themes and agenda was a group learning exercise that emphasized the need to progress and change the pipeline to lead to more successful and impactful careers in science, engineering, and medicine. He also described how the committee aimed to "conduct a workshop to present old information in a new way and develop new information that will hopefully change the success rate of Black men and Black women as they navigate their careers after they obtain degrees." Experiences as residents, fellows, and postdoctoral scientists are often dependent on the culture of the institution and leaders they encounter along the way, he noted, which is why it is important to look at individuals, institutions, and systems.

Co-chair Joan Y. Reede, M.D., M.P.H., M.S., M.B.A., Harvard Medical School, added her thanks to action group members, staff, and participants. She noted that the National Academies' report *Breaking Through: The Next Generation of Biomedical and Behavioral Science Researchers* (NASEM, 2018a) recognized that multiple sectors (e.g., government, education, industry, philanthropy, and accreditation bodies) involving intersecting systems must be engaged to effectively address workforce issues in the sciences. At the organizational level, academic medical centers, research enterprises, and associations are all involved. At the individual level, institutional leaders set policy, control finances, allocate resources, determine strategic directions, and have the ability to hold units and people accountable. In addition, individual actors within organizations serve as advisors, mentors, coaches, sponsors, and gatekeepers. She also took note of individual Black women and men who attempt to traverse what is often a lonely career path in order to transition from one level to another. They seek excellence with a desire to make meaningful contributions while addressing challenging environments hampered by inadequate resources and narrow professional networks. These are the same Black men and women, she added, who are also giving their time and effort in helping others move forward.

Publications from the National Academies including *The Impacts of Racism and Bias on Black People Pursuing Careers in Science, Engineering, and Medicine: Proceedings of a Workshop* (NASEM, 2020a) and *Promising Practices for Addressing the Underrepresentation of Women in Science, Engineering, and Medicine* (NASEM, 2020b) document bias, discrimination, and racism and experiences of harassment, marginalization, and microaggressions,

Dr. Reede pointed out. She said this workshop acknowledges the need for a forum to explore further what does and does not work in mentoring. She emphasized that while the need to address the entry and success of Black women and men into medical and graduate studies is clear, only achieving entry and graduation is not adequate. "We must improve the arc of representation at all levels," Dr. Reede stated. "To use a metaphor, it is important not only to have a seat but also to have a voice at the table, setting the table, determining the agenda, and inviting others to the table. Black men and women are needed in leadership."

ORGANIZATION OF THIS PROCEEDINGS

This publication summarizes the workshop *Mentoring and Advising of Black Students in Science, Engineering, and Medicine*. After introductory remarks highlighted in this chapter, Chapter 2 provides a summary of presentations on the current status of Black professionals in science and industry, with a focus on academic medicine and engineering. In Chapter 3, two medical school deans and an engineering college president offered perspectives on the advancement and promotion of Black faculty. Three "dyads" of mentors and mentees shared how their relationships began and have evolved, followed by discussion among them, summarized in Chapter 4. Chapter 5 summarizes a couple of social science perspectives, and four specific programs are presented in Chapter 6. Chapter 7 highlights report-outs from the breakout groups around a series of directed questions, as well as concluding comments by the workshop co-chairs. The workshop agenda and biographical sketches of the presenters can be found in Appendixes A and B, respectively.

In accordance with the policies of the National Academies, workshop participants did not attempt to establish any conclusions or recommendations about needs and future directions. In addition, the planning committee's role was limited to planning the workshop. This proceedings was prepared by the rapporteurs as a factual summary of what occurred at the workshop.

REFERENCES

NASEM (National Academies of Sciences, Engineering, and Medicine). 2018a. *Breaking Through: The Next Generation of Biomedical and Behavioral Science Researchers*. Washington, DC: The National Academies Press.

NASEM. 2018b. *An American Crisis: The Growing Absence of Black Men in Medicine and Science: Proceedings of a Joint Workshop*. Washington, DC: The National Academies Press.

NASEM. 2019. *The Science of Effective Mentorship in STEMM*. Washington, DC: The National Academies Press.

NASEM. 2020a. *The Impacts of Racism and Bias on Black People Pursuing Careers in Science, Engineering, and Medicine: Proceedings of a Workshop*. Washington, DC: The National Academies Press.

NASEM. 2020b. *Promising Practices for Addressing the Underrepresentation of Women in Science, Engineering, and Medicine*. Washington, DC: The National Academies Press.

2

Understanding the Current Status of Black Professionals in Academia and Industry

Highlights from the Presentation

- The percentages of Black faculty, department chairs, and deans in U.S. medical schools have stagnated, despite increases in the overall size of medical faculties (Dr. Poll-Hunter).
- Increasing representation will involve not just acting, but acting differently, including the infusing of a mentoring culture in a systems-based way (Dr. Poll-Hunter).
- A small study showed that African Americans enrolled in engineering who are part of the supportive ecosystem like the National Society of Black Engineers are 10 times more likely to graduate (Dr. Reid).
- Identity is a critical component of self-efficacy, which is affected by environment, personal factors, and behavior. A missing element is a sense of identity related to race, gender, and sexual orientation (Dr. Reid).

Randall C. Morgan Jr., M.D., M.B.A., Cobb/NMA Health Institute, moderated the first session to provide context for the discussions over the next 2 days. Norma Poll-Hunter, Ph.D., Association of American Medical Colleges (AAMC), shared data on medical school faculty and leadership to challenge the group to consider how to increase representation. Karl W.

Reid, Ed.D., National Society of Black Engineers (NSBE), shared insights from NSBE and research about the science, technology, engineering, and mathematics (STEM) pipeline and strategies to support high-achieving African American students.

BLACK FACULTY AND LEADERS AT VARIOUS STAGES OF TRANSITION

Dr. Poll-Hunter provided a statistical view of Black representation in U.S. medical schools, drawing primarily on AAMC data. Blacks/African Americans represented 6.2 percent of medical school graduates in 2018–2019. They were 5.1 percent of residents, 5.0 percent of active U.S. physicians, and 3.6 percent of full-time medical school (M.D.) faculty. Looking more closely at 2019 faculty data, there were 6,503 Black/African American faculty members out of 179,238 faculty members in total. (An additional 511 individuals reported mixed Black and other race/ethnicity.) By rank, the breakdown was as follows:

- Full professor: 755
- Associate professor: 1,202
- Assistant professor: 3,748
- Instructor: 664
- Other: 134

By sex, Black women were 2.1 percent of all full-time faculty; Black men were 1.5 percent of full-time faculty. Looked at another way, women were 58.5 percent of the total among full-time Black faculty. Rank-wise, Black women were 5.8 percent of assistant, 4.5 percent of associate, and 2.8 percent of full professors. Black men were 3.3 percent of assistant, 2.46 percent of associate, and 1.6 percent of full professors. "When we look across faculty ranks for all underrepresented minorities, the representation decreases going up faculty rank," she commented. "There is a lot of work to be done here."

Looking at faculty by both gender and race and ethnicity, the percentage has been stagnant from 2010 to 2019, despite the growth of medical school faculties overall. "The work that you are doing here today is going to be really critical in changing the course and trajectory from this point forward," she said to workshop participants. She called attention to AAMC data (Liu and Morrison, 2014) on retention and attrition statistics for new assistant professors entering faculties in institutions in 2000. Although the data are older, Dr. Poll-Hunter singled out two points: (1) Black or African American faculty are likely to leave academia and (2) they leave sooner and at a faster rate than other population groups.

Looking further along the career trajectory, she shared data about department chairs by discipline and ethnicity. Across medical school faculties, there were 3,297 department chairs in 2019, of whom 120 were Black, or 3.6 percent of all chairs. Black faculty were 4 percent of clinical science department chairs and 2.2 percent of basic science department chairs. Related to medical school deans, publicly available AAMC data are disaggregated as underrepresented minorities (URM) or non-underrepresented minorities (not by specific race/ethnicity) and also as serving in a permanent or interim/acting capacity. In 1990, URMs were 6 percent of permanent deans (no interim/acting URM deans). In 2010, there were 10 percent URM permanent deans and 22 percent interim/acting deans. In 2019, the permanent number was the same at 10 percent, and the percentage of interim/acting had decreased to 16 percent. "This tells us there are opportunities, but we need to do a better job, especially with individuals who are in the pipeline as interim and acting deans to support them to get to that next stage of attaining permanent step. We have a pipeline of leaders, but they are not making it to that next step," she said.

Dr. Poll-Hunter said her intention in sharing the data was not only to act, but to act *differently*. Based on what is known (e.g., Harris et al., 2018; Sanchez, 2020), she said, mentorship and sponsorship are beneficial, but not everyone has access to this kind of support. She raised several questions, including these two:

1. How can we decrease reliance on person-dependent solutions and consider other strategies to infuse a culture of mentoring in a systems-based way?
2. How can we make information about the pathway to success from pre-faculty to full professorship more transparent and accessible?

Person-to-person programs are critical, she clarified, but she suggested finding ways to expand the number of people reached. She noted the concept of "pre-faculty" as a concept to attract Black individuals and other URMs to careers in academic medicine by providing tools and the "playbook" to get into academia. She also suggested applying practices that work at other points of the continuum, such as holistic reviews (Harris et al., 2018) used for medical school student recruitment, to increase faculty diversity. In conclusion, she asked, "How can we foster inclusive, anti-racism institutional cultures and climate to facilitate faculty thriving?"

ENGINEERING PERSPECTIVE

Dr. Reid reinforced the questions posed by Dr. Poll-Hunter and said he would focus on the early stages of the pipeline. "We cannot produce faculty professionals if they are not proficient in math and science in fourth and eighth grades," he stated. "These early milestones matter." He noted some of these issues were being discussed when he was an engineering undergraduate at the Massachusetts Institute of Technology (MIT) 30 years ago. "It is time to foster systemic change," he stressed, adding that "engineers look at challenges systemically."

While working at the United Negro College Fund, Dr. Reid asked the Frederick D. Patterson Research Institute to look at where people are falling outside of educational pathways by focusing on children who were ages 0 to 5 at the time of the 2010 census and who could be heading through high school and college later in the decade. The data showed a lower percentage of Latinx and especially Black children made it through to college graduation:

- Among white children (ages 0 to 5 in 2010, 2,622,787 in total), 85 percent completed high school; of those who completed high school, 67 percent enrolled in college; of those, 62 percent graduated in 6 years. Overall, 35 percent in this cohort graduated from college in 10 years.
- Among Latinx children (ages 0 to 5 in 2010, 986,657 in total), 76 percent completed high school; of those, 69 percent enrolled in college; of those, 51 percent graduated in 6 years. Overall, 27 percent of this cohort graduated from college in 10 years.
- Among African American children (ages 0 to 5 in 2010, 568,211 in total), 68 percent completed high school; of those who graduated high school, 62 percent enrolled in college; of those, 40 percent graduated within 6 years. Overall, 16 percent in this cohort graduated college in 10 years, and only 10 percent in low-income communities.

Looking at STEM among all racial and ethnic groups, data from the National Center for Educational Statistics reveal that the "STEM pipeline is leaking badly," as Dr. Reid said. From a cohort of 4,012,770 ninth-graders in 2001, 70 percent graduated high school in 2005, and 1,303,050 were college-ready in fall of 2005. Of this number, 21 percent majored in a STEM discipline, but there was an attrition rate of 60 percent. Thus, the group of more than 4 million ninth-graders produced 166,530 STEM graduates by 2011, or only 4 percent of the total. A major drop-off point occurred among students who planned to major in a STEM discipline but did not complete these majors.

Dr. Reid participated in an Association of Public Land Grant Universities comprehensive analysis of diversity in engineering education (APLU, 2018). Overall, it showed a 42 percent increase in bachelor's degrees in engineering awarded between 2010–2011 and 2015–2016. The number of Black students increased by 35 percent, and there was a 79 percent increase in Hispanic students graduating with engineering degrees. Despite the percentage increases, he noted that the overall number remained low, and only 3.9 percent of engineering degrees awarded went to Black students. At the master's level, 2 percent of engineering degrees went to Black students. At the doctoral level, the overall increase was 36 percent, but the number is extremely low, with 1.9 percent of all doctoral degrees awarded to Black students.

Gender is another challenge in engineering. "We're leaving a lot of talent on the table," he said. Although Black women earn the overall majority of all bachelor's degrees awarded to African Americans, they earn only 24.9 percent of engineering bachelor's degrees compared with Black men. Likewise, Black women earn 69.6 percent of all master's degrees awarded to Black students, but 28.2 percent of engineering master's degrees.

Dr. Reid said NSBE can play a role in boosting graduation rates. As an overview, NSBE has about 22,000 members, largely undergraduates in more than 300 accredited engineering programs. There is also a pre-collegiate program with about 4,200 practicing engineers and about 3,650 professional members. A small study (Ross and McGrade, 2016) showed that African Americans enrolled in engineering who are part of the NSBE ecosystem are 10 times more likely to graduate than those who are not involved.

One reason for this outcome, he said, stems from his own research on factors contributing to African American success in higher education, adapted from the social cognitive theory of Albert Bandura (1997). Bandura posited that self-efficacy is affected by environment, personal factors, and behavior; all three must be attended to, rather than any one of them in iso-

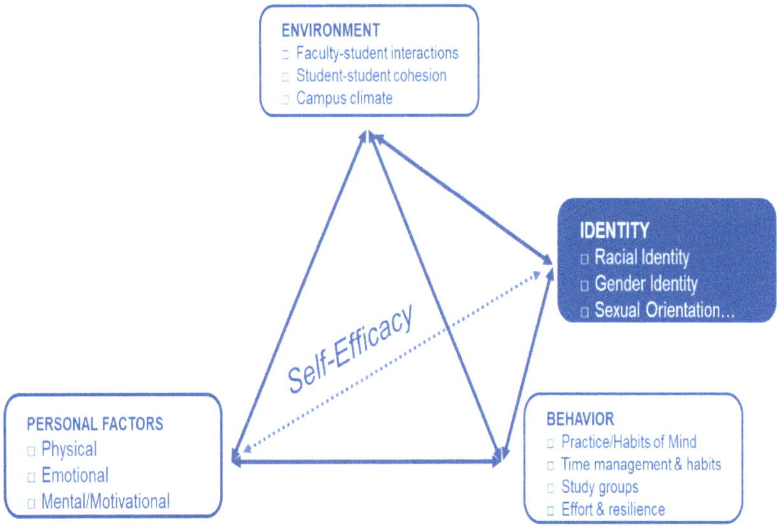

FIGURE 2-1 A modified social cognitive framework to identify factors for African American student success.
SOURCE: Karl Reid, Workshop Presentation, December 7, 2020, adapted from Bandura, 1997.

lation for a successful outcome. Dr. Reid said he argued in his dissertation that a missing element is a sense of identity related to race, gender, and sexual orientation (see Figure 2-1). He described the outcomes of his study to explain what matters for high-achieving Black males in college also applies to workforce. These factors included (1) high confidence in their academic ability; (2) strong "vertical" relationships with faculty; (3) social integration on campus in "horizontal relationships"; and (4) strong internalized racial identity.

NSBE has worked with other organizations to scale up success to create the "50K Coalition" with a goal to produce 50,000 female, Hispanic, Native American, and Black engineers annually by 2025.[1] Other NSBE resources include a white paper with engagement strategies (Reid et al., 2016), a student retention toolkit, and a "collaborative roadmap" with the Society of Women Engineers and the Women in Engineering ProActive Network that focuses on African American women in undergraduate engineering.

[1] See https://50kcoalition.org/.

DISCUSSION

Dr. Morgan asked Dr. Poll-Hunter to comment on Dr. Reid's idea of identity in accounting for the success of African American students. She replied that Bandura's framework, which she used in her own dissertation in the South Bronx, shows ways to persist in times of stress. Role models and positive reinforcement can be replicated at a systems level to help Black men and women persist and be successful, she said.

In response to a question about academic engineers, Dr. Reid said when he served as an associate dean at MIT, data showed that 92 percent of incoming URMs said they wanted to attend graduate school, but 5 years later, very few enrolled at the master's and Ph.D. levels. Using social cognitive theory to determine what explains the gap, he and others looked at how to create both vertical (with faculty) and horizontal (with peers on campus) connections. A program began in 2006 with a cohort of about 25 freshmen and sophomores who expressed interest in graduate education and "stayed with them" for 3.5 years. Modeled after the Ronald E. McNair Scholars Program,[2] the group met monthly, conducted research, attended conferences, and had opportunities to make presentations. The program continues today, and Black graduate enrollment grew from about 5 to 13 percent.

NSBE also partners with the Academic and Research Leadership Network, founded at Georgia Tech, and offers an academic track at its annual conventions. A National Science Foundation grant helps send postdoctoral scholars and early-career faculty to the conference.

REFERENCES

APLU (Association of Public and Land Grant Universities). 2018. *The 2018 Status Report on Engineering Education: A Snapshot of Diversity in Degrees Conferred in Engineering.* https://www.aplu.org/library/the-2018-status-report-on-engineering-education-a-snapshot-of-diversity-in-degrees-conferred-in-engineering.

Bandura, A. 1997. *Self-Efficacy: The Exercise of Control.* New York: W. H. Freeman and Company.

Harris, T. B., W. A. Thomson, N. P. Moreno, S. Conrad, S. E. White, G. H. Young, E. D Malmberg, B. Weisman, and A. D. H. Monroe. 2018. Advancing holistic review for faculty recruitment and advancement. *Academic Medicine* 93(11): 1658–1662.

Liu, C., and E. Morrison. 2014. *U.S. Medical School Full-time Faculty Attrition.* AAMC. Analysis in Brief, Vol. 14(2).

[2] See https://mcnairscholars.com/about.

Reid, K., M. Ross, and N. Yates. 2016. *Paving the Way: Institutional Interventions for Academic Excellence and Success in Engineering.* https://diversityrecognition.asee.org/wp-content/uploads/sites/22/2019/03/Paving-the-Way-NSBE-White-Paper-Reid-Ross-Yates-Resource.pdf.

Ross, M., and S. McGrade. 2016. An Exploration into the Impacts of the National Society of Black Engineers (NSBE) on Student Persistence. Presentation. 123rd ASEE Annual Conference and Exposition, June 26–29, 2016.

Sanchez, J. (ed.). 2020. *Succeeding in Academic Medicine: A Roadmap for Diverse Medical Students and Residents.* Cham, Switzerland: Springer International Publishing.

3

Ensuring the Advancement and Promotion of Black Faculty

Highlights from the Presentations

- Harvard Medical School has four goals in its Better Together Plan to cultivate an environment of inclusiveness and collaboration: (1) developing people and infrastructure, (2) building community and belonging, (3) addressing culture and communication, and (4) ensuring accountability and generating new knowledge (Dr. Daley).
- Guiding principles have been established to consider Harvard Medical School's 238-year history in the context of current-day spaces, artwork, and commemoration of individuals in an effort to promote a more inclusive campus (Dr. Daley).
- In the first year of a program to provide debt-free education to Weill Cornell Medicine students with financial need, more underrepresented minorities, participants in the American Association of Medical Colleges Fee Assistance program, and graduates of public universities enrolled, with no drop in medical exam scores (Dr. Choi).
- An important aspect of enhancing diversity and inclusion is engaging across an "ecosystem" that includes students, faculty, administrators, and the board of directors and donors (Dr. Choi).
- False assumptions, or myths, used to justify the underrepresentation of Black people in science and engineering

include a shortage of talent, that a meritocracy prevails, and that diversity automatically results in inclusion (Dr. Barabino).
- As articulated by psychologist Kecia Thomas, "pet to threat" describes the situation when junior faculty members of color are initially doted upon, then maligned when they start to accomplish and threaten the existing system (Dr. Barabino).

MaCalus V. Hogan, M.D., M.B.A., University of Pittsburgh Medical Center, moderated a session that was comprised of two medical school deans and the president of a college of engineering: George Q. Daley, M.D., Ph.D., Harvard Medical School; Augustine C. K. Choi, M.D., Weill Cornell Medicine; and Gilda A. Barabino, Ph.D., Olin College of Engineering. Dr. Hogan noted he himself is a mentee of workshop co-chair Randall Morgan and Roundtable chair Cato Laurencin, which he commented speaks to the power of mentoring.

HARVARD MEDICAL SCHOOL

Dr. Daley spoke about efforts at Harvard Medical School (HMS) to have a faculty that reflects the diversity of the patients served across the HMS system, including in affiliate hospitals. In late 2016, after his appointment as dean was announced but before he began, he identified diversity as one of his core priorities. It is central to, and written into, the strategic plan and mission statement.

To focus this effort, Dr. Daley constituted a task force chaired by Dr. Joan Reede, dean for diversity and community partnership, comprised of 36 administrators, staff, faculty, postdocs, and students. The task force recommended a comprehensive plan to convert HMS to become an institution of preference for candidates from diverse backgrounds. Four key goals were articulated: (1) developing people and infrastructure, (2) building community and belonging, (3) addressing culture and communication, and (4) ensuring accountability and generating new knowledge. This is the basis of the school's Better Together Plan.[1]

The task force issued announcements throughout the process, with release of a comprehensive report in June 2020. Although coincidental,

[1] See https://hms.harvard.edu/about-hms/campus-culture/diversity-inclusion/better-together-plan.

the timing was all the more meaningful in the context of national actions against racism, Dr. Daley observed. He noted,

> Recognizing the challenges in a society that aspires to justice and fairness but falls short, deep societal rifts will not be alleviated by a short campaign. We at HMS have been dedicated to a longer-term struggle. Some days, I am overwhelmed at what needs to be done, but some days I am filled with hope as I see the steps we are taking.

In 2019, he and Dr. Reede held a series of meetings with affiliate hospitals' CEOs and other senior leaders. "We put on the table the grim realities of the lack of progress we have made in representation in our faculty," he said. "We challenged them to partner with us, both in recruiting and advancing URiM [underrepresented in medicine] faculty." Harvard has the largest medical school in the nation, with 11,000 faculty members mostly working in affiliate hospitals. Eleven percent are full professors, 14 percent are associate professors, and most of the rest are assistant professors and instructors. Between January 2018 and September 2020, 82 URiM faculty were promoted: 57 to assistant, 16 to associate, and 7 to full professor. While the numbers are promising, progress must continue, he acknowledged. He and Dr. Reede have asked department heads to focus on URiM leadership opportunities. In the past year, three URiM faculty have been named to leadership positions in the affiliate hospitals: Nawal Nour, M.D., M.P.H.; Edward Rodriquez, M.D., Ph.D.; and Seun Johnson-Akeju, M.D. A virtual dinner was held to celebrate these promotions, and the three leaders shared their experiences. "We build strength by coming together as a community, supporting one another, and celebrating successes," Dr. Daley commented.

HMS is also committed to supporting affinity groups, such as a new Black Postdoctoral Association and a Black Staff Caucus. Another new initiative focuses on the core basic science departments. In the last 10 faculty searches, excellent URiM candidates were not selected because of a focus on narrow scientific subspecialties. To counter the focus on scientific fit, he and department chairs launched what they call a cluster hire, which allows for hiring up to four positions in one round of recruitment. In addition to exceptional scholarship, they seek candidates who have a demonstrated commitment to the mission and values that include advancing diversity and inclusiveness. In the applicant pool of 680 applications to date for the cluster hires, at least 130 are from URiM candidates.

According to Dr. Daley, these efforts have inspired the affiliates to launch similar searches. The Office for Faculty Affairs is making meaningful strides to recognize dedication to diversity and inclusion as part of the promotions process. The Harvard CV template is being revised to reflect achievements in advancing diversity and anti-racism.

A committee on artwork and cultural representation is promoting a more inclusive climate on campus. Public works of art now include a portrait of Dr. William Augustus Hinton, the school's first Black full professor. As an institution that is 238 years old, Harvard Medical School is steeped in history, Dr. Daley noted, but also must "recognize the missteps." Guiding principles have been established to consider the school's history, spaces, artwork, and how to commemorate individuals. Applying these principles, a student society named for Oliver Wendell Holmes (who admitted the first Black students in 1850 but expelled them the next year after white students and faculty protested) was renamed for Dr. Hinton.

"As scientists and physicians, we are constantly reviewing and critiquing to ensure we are making progress in our aspirations of social justice," Dr. Daley said. He stressed the importance of being able to safely discuss mistakes in order to move forward and learn. A statement of mutual respect and public discourse (HMS, 2021) frames and guides discussions about such issues as diversity in clinical research, being a first-generation college student, the imposter syndrome, and microaggressions. Specialized fellowships, such as the Commonwealth Fund Fellowship in Minority Health (see Chapter 6 for information about this program), are preparing physicians, especially URiM physicians, to become leaders to transform health-care delivery systems, health equity, and the social determinants of health.

Dr. Daley concluded that it is critical to celebrate diversity and chart a course for improvement so the HMS community can nurture the best science, education, and service. "We need to remedy the pipeline problem in the biomedical and other STEM [science, technology, engineering, and mathematics] fields, interface better with patients and communities, and reduce health disparities," he said, because "faculty are the cornerstone of Harvard Medical School."

WEILL CORNELL MEDICINE

Dr. Choi discussed ongoing, new, and developing strategies to ensure the advancement and promotion of Black faculty at Weill Cornell Medicine (WCM). These strategies aim to enhance the culture of equity and belonging, strengthen the pipeline, focus on faculty recruitment, optimize mentorship and career development, and engage board leadership and donors.

Current faculty composition is about 55 percent men and 45 percent women, Dr. Choi said. By race and ethnicity, "the numbers are not as good as we want them to be": The faculty is 64 percent Caucasian, 28 percent Asian, and 7 percent URiM. In the past 4 or 5 years, resources have been invested to move the needle on faculty development. From 2016 to 2020, overall faculty numbers grew 16 percent (from 1,649 to 1,908). URiM faculty increased by 47 percent (from 111 to 163), and women faculty increased by 21 percent (from 721 to 874). Most are at the junior faculty level, especially assistant professors, and he said improvement is needed at all levels.

He said enhancing the culture of equity and belonging requires top-down, bottom-up, and peer-led efforts. The diversity dean sits on the Dean's Leadership Council, and there are also two associate and two assistant deans for diversity. All departments hold seminars during the school's Diversity Week. Other recent initiatives include WCM strategic planning to include diversity, Dean's Diversity and Healthcare Disparity Research Awards, and governance through a newly formed Office of Institutional Equity. All faculty, staff, and students must complete anti-bias training, which he characterized at the 101 (basic) level with plans for 102 (more advanced) training in early 2021. Proactive efforts also include an anti-racism task force launched in 2020 and senior-level diversity champions in every department. There are also a number of Weill/Cornell pipeline programs from middle and high schools through college, medical/graduate school, and residency/postdoctoral to academic leaders.

Last year, funds were raised to launch a debt-free scholarship program, in perpetuity, for students with financial need. It covers all costs of attendance, not just tuition. Preliminary analysis of incoming 2020 students shows a significant increase of URiM students (from about 21 to 29 percent), American Association of Medical Colleges Fee Assistance program participants, and graduates of public universities compared with the previous 3 years, with no change in academic scores.

New programs are also aiming to transition to residents at the WCM Medical Center and then to WCM faculty positions, and to retaining WCM postdoctoral scholars as faculty. A linkage with City University of New York–Hunter College, as part of the Clinical and Translational Science Center, is being deepened, and a new relationship with a Historically Black College and University (HBCU) medical college is under development, Dr. Choi said.

Faculty recruitment prioritizes diversity as a marker of institutional excellence. It is built into the search committee process policies, and a program is being developed to support departments in recruiting diverse faculty. Mentoring and faculty development are important for all faculty, especially for URiM faculty, Dr. Choi said. A Mentoring Academy was established in 2018 to foster mentorship and sponsoring across career pathways. JumpStart Research Career Development, launched in 2019, provides seed funds to senior postdoctoral scholars and junior faculty to help in the transition to become independent scientists. Relaunched in 2020, Research Assistance for Primary Parents provides technical assistance to faculty who are primary caretakers of their children.

It is important to engage board leadership and donors, Dr. Choi said. There is now a Board Special Committee on Equity, Diversity and Inclusion that charges the board to advance initiatives in equity, diversity, and inclusion at WCM and in the delivery of health care. Dr. Choi stressed the "Equity and Social Justice ecosystem" consists of the range of groups and efforts at the student, faculty, staff, leadership, and board levels. "We want to continue to move the needle as a society and at Weill Cornell Medicine," he said.

OLIN COLLEGE OF ENGINEERING

Dr. Barabino spoke more broadly about the advancement and promotion of Black faculty. She reminded participants that Black people make up 13 percent of the U.S. population but only 5 percent of faculty across all disciplines and 4 percent of new Ph.D.s in science and engineering, which undermines the health and well-being of the nation. The gap persists despite years-long interventions such as future faculty programs, fellowships, visiting professorships, professional development programs, and more.

To understand the reasons, she urged a focus on social-organizational factors that are institutional, environmental, and structural and that are deeply embedded and often overlooked. "The system needs to change, and we can start by challenging assumptions, also known as myths," she stated. These assumptions include a presumed shortage of talent, presumed meritocracy, and a presumed link between diversity and inclusion. Related to presumed shortage of talent, although the numbers are low, there are many talented Black engineers and scientists from whom to draw, she said. The assumption of meritocracy can perpetuate inequities, reinforce privilege, and provide a convenient excuse for biased and unfair behavior.

She also challenged as false the assumption that inclusion automatically accompanies diversity.

Real change requires an inclusive culture, Dr. Barabino said. Creating an inclusive culture requires acceptance of the authenticity of the message, open dialogue followed by meaningful action, equitable adherence to policies and practices, recognition of scholarly contributions and behind-the-scenes contributions (sometimes referred to as a "cultural tax"), deep respect for cultures and cultural competence, and a proactive stance on righting wrongs. HBCUs can provide lessons, she said. HBCUs provide valuable examples for creating inclusive environments. She referred to her alma mater, Xavier University of Louisiana, as an example. Xavier has been described as a place that "nurtures its students and feeds their souls" with an emphasis on excellence, a supportive community, and leadership. Students are expected to succeed, and alignment of professional and racial identity go hand in hand. As important as discipline-based knowledge, she noted,

> Socialization is critical for career advancement: that is, understanding the ways of practicing, understanding unwritten rules and norms, and understanding how to navigate the system. As you can imagine, this requires coaching from those already in the system.

Dr. Barabino and social scientist Dr. Cheryl Leggon led a research-driven project to unpack factors involved in the careers of minority women in academic engineering (Leggon and Barabino, 2015). Lessons learned include the importance of mentors, sponsors, and champions; the importance of communalism (free exchange of ideas), community, and community building to create a sense of belonging; and the importance of contextual and longitudinal data disaggregated by race/ethnicity and gender.

Beyond socialization, strategies to promote career advancement include recognition, informed and culturally competent faculty and administrators, and new models and styles of mentoring and advocacy, recognizing that there is no one-size-fits-all. "Leaders who are not of color often make assumptions about whether or not the person who does not look like them has been afforded the same networking and mentoring opportunities to advance their careers," she observed. "They and all leaders must be open to learning and acting in ways that are supportive." While same-race/same-gender mentoring is desirable, the dearth of minority faculty does not always make this possible. "We don't necessarily have to have mentors and advocates from the same backgrounds, but we do need to have mentors and advocates who understand the experiences, and we need leaders who hold themselves and others in their organizations accountable," she observed. She also called for adjusted evaluation and reward systems, as well as restructured environments that ensure inclusivity and provide a supportive community for progression and for functional mentoring, networking, and collaboration.

Black faculty must navigate at the intersection of competence and authority, she said. They are often hypervisible when it comes to service and invisible when it comes to recognition and inclusion in collaborations or having their work cited. She also warned about a concept called "pet to threat," described by Kecia Thomas (Thomas et al., 2013), in which junior faculty of color are embraced when first hired and given development opportunities but seen as tokens; then, when they start to excel, are perceived as upsetting the status quo by outperforming majority colleagues and as undeserving of awards or success. Their competence is often met with hostility, which impedes career progress.

Career advancement is attainable when these factors are addressed. "Black talent abounds," she concluded. "Current and future Black leaders are ready. I invite everyone to join us."

DISCUSSION

A participant commented on the MARC (Minority Access to Research Careers) Scholars funded by the National Institutes of Health. However well prepared the students are, they have not been accepted by Ph.D. programs or are advised to do a postbac program first at a higher rate than other students. Dr. Choi said he planned to look at the data related to MARC Scholars at his institution.

Dr. Hogan asked the participants what they see as the main challenges to promotion for Black and Latinx faculty and how to overcome the hurdles. Dr. Daley noted retention and promotion is a broad problem among all academic medicine faculty, but disproportionately occurs for faculty who are women and faculty of color. "We need targeted sponsorship programs that identify individuals as future leaders and target unique and empowering support to them," he said, citing Harvard's Commonwealth Fund Fellowship program in Minority Health Policy as an example.[2] He continued, "We are also learning as a community that mentorship does not mean color-blind mentorship. It means targeted, unique strategies

[2] For more information, see https://cff.hms.harvard.edu/.

for supporting the needs of the scholars in our community." A train-the-trainer model now provides better training about mentorship that speaks to the needs of the Black faculty. With the largest medical school faculty in the country, there are more than 600 faculty of color in the HMS system. "What we really need to do is continue to increase representation. We must create a safe haven community within community by bringing our physicians and scientific scholars of color together," he said.

Dr. Barabino said many challenges to promotion are invisible, but they accumulate. "Biases, slights, challenges to authority, not being included in collaboration, these go unnoticed and unnamed," she said. "They need to be made visible to talk about them." She gave such examples as how criteria for success are set up, who is setting them up, and the subjectivity of evaluations. "It is cumulative, it wears people down over time but holds them back." Courageous leadership, she pointed out, does not always translate and get put into action.

Dr. Daley referred to the observation by Dr. Barabino about having a system that recognizes microaggressions and provides remediation. A few years ago, he said, Harvard recognized that medical students, especially in the surgical subspecialties, were suffering mistreatment in many areas, including related to racism. A learning environment review was instituted in which students anonymously reported their experiences in their clinical clerkships, and the data were aggregated and shown to departments. "What we have seen is slow uptick in improved reporting from students," he said. As learned from patient safety and quality improvement, feedback cannot be presented in a judgmental way with shame. "Think of it as a 'Morbidity and Mortality Report' for racism," he said. "We need to be able to recognize our mistakes but have a blame-free culture of continuous improvement."

Dr. Choi agreed with the top-down, bottom-up, and peer-led strategies discussed by Dr. Daley and Dr. Barabino. "It's about being color blind but also seeing color," he said.

> Oftentimes, I get asked about a metric of success beyond the numbers. To me, one intangible metric of success is we have to get to the point that when you see a microaggression or racist behavior, it goes to the level of intolerance as when we view child abuse.... We're not there yet. But during rounding in a hospital with an attending physician along with residents, interns, and students, if anyone sees a microaggression, they need to be able to get that issue

> to the right place and not look the other way. We as a community are not there yet, but I think we are gearing toward that, and I think that is quite important.

Dr. Hogan asked about mentorship in scientific environments outside of hospitals and other medical settings. Dr. Barabino responded that the environment in which people are trained is important. Many students start out in a STEM field, often with the desire to give back to their communities, but they feel pushed out and leave. "We should provide an environment to show them how to excel," she said. "Matching up goals with the environment that allows them to meet those goals will make a difference." Instead, gatekeepers push people out. They need to understand the messages sent by their behaviors, such as through disparaging comments, not making eye contact in the classroom, or choosing how the institution represents itself.

Medicine and STEM in general are hard, added Dr. Daley, and it is a toil and travail to get through the schooling and training. Loss of research funding is a further challenge. "We have to recognize the challenges but also take steps to make careers in science and medicine more appealing for everyone, but in particular for those communities who are already underrepresented," he said. He reiterated Dr. Barabino's point about the need for role models so people facing these challenging fields can look up and can "see themselves" in outstanding leaders.

Dr. Choi noted his institution has an Office of Diversity and Inclusion. A sense of belonging is essential, but not a given. He disagrees with the assertion by some people that diversity and inclusion must be achieved before belonging can occur. "We need to achieve belonging and we are not there yet," he said. "The sense of belonging is critical. What does it mean? It means we value what you say. It means, you will help us get better. That is our goal." Culture is powerful, he added. "We have to get to a culture of equity." He also commented that while the appointment of a person of color as a dean of diversity to sit on WCM's leadership council was important, more people took note when the new dean of admissions named was a person of color.

Dr. Hogan thanked the presenters and asked the workshop co-chairs for additional comments. Dr. Reede reflected on both sessions so far. She noted it began with a grounding of the data by Dr. Poll-Hunter and Dr. Reid (see Chapter 2). Hearing from the leaders in this session showed movement from words of support for diversity to actions. "I am witnessing the growth of our leaders and what they see," she said. "I heard many wonderful ideas to carry this work forward and a clear message of intentionality, transparency, and accountability. We have been involved in these conversations for many years. We don't need to repeat the same conversations, but need to move forward."

Dr. Morgan noted when he and Dr. Reede planned the workshop, they agreed it could not cover the entire pipeline. This robust discussion proves the need to focus on academic institutions and transition points, and the role that one or two people can make in a person's career. Creating the environment where people can belong is extremely important, and HBCUs also provide valuable lessons, he added.

REFERENCES

HMS (Harvard Medical School). 2021. Statement of Mutual Respect and Discourse at HMS. https://hms.harvard.edu/about-hms/campus-culture/statement-mutual-respect-public-discourse-hms.

Leggon, C., and G. Barabino. 2015. Socializing African American female engineers into academic careers: The case of the cross-disciplinary initiative for minority women faculty. Chapter 9 in J. B. Slaughter, Y. Tao, and W. Pearson, Jr. (eds.), *Changing the Face of Engineering: The African American Experience*. Baltimore: Johns Hopkins University Press.

Thomas, K. M., J. Johnson-Bailey, R. E. Phelps, N. M. Tran, and L. Johnson. 2013. Moving from pet to threat: Narratives of professional Black women. In L. Comas-Diaz and B. Green (eds.), *The Psychological Health of Women of Color*. Westport, CT: Praeger.

4

Mentor-Mentee Conversations

Highlights from the Presentations

- A mentor-mentee relationship does not suddenly happen. Sometimes another person needs to facilitate the connection to allow the "magic" to happen (Dr. Dzirasa and Dr. Allsop).
- Mentors and mentees do not have to be at the same institution or the same physical space to have a strong relationship (Dr. Dzirasa and Dr. Allsop).
- Sponsors and mentors provide different benefits, but both types of relationships must be built on communication and follow-up (Dr. Higginbotham and Dr. Ross).
- The mentee or person being sponsored needs to prioritize the time needed for the relationship, act on the suggestions or connections made, and provide feedback about the results of the interactions to the mentor or sponsor (Dr. Higginbotham and Dr. Ross).
- A successful relationship is built on shared vision and values (Dr. Barabino and Dr. Banton).
- Mentoring is a two-way street; the mentor will also learn and benefit from the relationship (Dr. Barabino and Dr. Banton).

This session was set up as three sets of free-form conversations between long-standing mentors and mentees: Kafui Dzirasa, M.D., Ph.D., Duke University, and Aza Allsop, M.D., Ph.D., Yale University; Eve Higginbotham, S.M., M.D., University of Pennsylvania, and Ahmara Ross, M.D., Ph.D., University of Pennsylvania; and Gilda Barabino, Ph.D., Olin College of Engineering, and Shereka Banton, Ph.D., Johnson & Johnson. Session moderator Wendy Yallowitz, M.S.W., Robert Wood Johnson Foundation, introduced the session by explaining the pairs would discuss how their relationships began and changed over time, challenges in the interactions, best practices, and lessons learned.

CONVERSATIONS WITH LONG-STANDING MENTORS AND MENTEES

Kafui Dzirasa, M.D., Ph.D., and Aza Allsop, M.D., Ph.D.

Dr. Allsop recounted the first meeting with his mentor Dr. Dzirasa at a Gordon Research Conference and seeing "this other Black guy working on a presentation." Later, Dr. Dzirasa came to Dr. Allsop's poster session to discuss it with him. "There was a resonance in the way he thought about the science," Dr. Allsop recalled. "We started talking about our stories, it was affirming for me that this [career] is attainable and doable. And I can still be cool and attain it."

Dr. Dzirasa added to the picture. He noted he is often the only or one of the only Black participants at a scientific meeting. In addition, Dr. Allsop's Ph.D. advisor had asked Dr. Dzirasa to reach out to her advisee at the poster session, recognizing the importance of Dr. Allsop connecting with another Black man physician-scientist. Thus, Dr. Dzirasa said, in terms of a best practice, sometimes someone else has to take the initiative to make the connection. "So often we take for granted the magic that is supposed to randomly happen when two people come together, when the 'magic' was totally planned out by his Ph.D. advisor," he said.

Dr. Dzirasa added that he has experienced failures, such as grants not won, and "for me, the most important part of mentoring him is get the losses into the win column." He elaborated on this point: "This person reminded me of myself. All those things they didn't fund me for, they will fund him for. There was an immediate instinct of creating a better version of myself. By that, I don't mean to turn him into me, but I want him not to have all the challenges and run into the same barriers that I did. How can I help him to go further?"

They were at different institutions, and their second encounter was a phone call. Dr. Allsop was navigating the significant transition for physician-scientists when they leave their labs and go to medical school. He asked Dr. Dzirasa for advice. "My project was at a point that if I could just do a little bit more, it could be a higher-impact paper. I was thinking of taking a year off to do a postdoc," he said. Dr. Dzirasa helped him map out a path and made the decision easier.

In helping Dr. Allsop navigate this major decision point for a physician-scientist, Dr. Dzirasa noted he was guided by advice from his own mentor who had previously challenged him to structure his own residency and research differently. "I was able to share how he [Dr. Allsop] could set himself up to have the best opportunities down the line. The postdoc capitalized on the research he was doing to extend his science product and also to navigate and negotiate for more research training later," Dr. Dzirasa said. "At every step, I could help him think through transitions relevant 2 or 3 years down the line."

They continued to meet and catch up at different meetings and conferences. Then, in what he described as "selfish motivations," he realized, "I should be recruiting him to come to Duke." Dr. Allsop did not ultimately go to Duke, but appreciated how Dr. Dzirasa "filled me up as much as possible with ego strength to prepare me to advocate for myself, no matter where I ended up." For example, Dr. Dzirasa told Dr. Allsop that he could start a lab while in residency and be successful. Dr. Allsop recalled that

> He [Dr. Dzirasa] served as an example and role model, and he shifted my framework. Part of being a great mentor is being willing to be vulnerable and really share failures and the successes, and all the factors—the stresses—that come along with that. He shared how difficult it was, too.

With Dr. Dzirasa's guidance, Dr. Allsop developed a "game plan" and negotiated an independent research and residency program. He appreciated how Dr. Dzirasa balanced advice, friendship, and recognition that Dr. Allsop had to "find his own place," which meant "being generous about not putting recruitment before the relationship." To that, Dr. Dzirasa added, "I believe in being really honest and vulnerable about mentoring. I have had mentors who have tried to recruit me to different places, but I am not at any of those places. I made it very clear that he has the space to decide what is best for him." Ultimately, Dr. Allsop called him to tell him he would be going to Yale.

Dr. Dzirasa stressed the importance of having a mentor or other person offering positivity. "If you see a prize fighter, they always have a coach next to them saying they are the best fighter to ever walk into the earth," he commented. "I have had that at every stage of my career. It doesn't matter if it is true, it propels me to be the best version of myself. We will both continue to fail, but we will both continue to push the envelope."

Dr. Dzirasa also pointed out they have never been at the same institution. "The mentor-mentee relationship does not have to be contained within a physical setting." He noted that their relationship began as two Black scientists at a Gordon Research Conference and, several years later, when they were both in Boston for a conference, they did so as "two Black M.D./Ph.D. scientists celebrating the launch of a career."

Eve Higginbotham, S.M., M.D., and Ahmara Ross, M.D., Ph.D.

Dr. Higginbotham clarified that she considers herself to be Dr. Ross's sponsor more than mentor. She elaborated, "I look for opportunities for Dr. Ross to shine. It's about having her career at the top of mind at all times and determining in my own pathway what I can share with her and how I can leverage my decades of experience in ophthalmology to benefit her. As a sponsor, I am willing to put myself out publicly and endorse her, and I take the time to do that."

Dr. Ross explained that she originally planned to go into oncology but realized it was not a good fit when she was already well into her M.D./Ph.D. program. She enjoyed her ophthalmology rotation, especially using her clinical and research expertise to focus on glaucoma, where she realized she could make a difference for patients of color. Her mentor, Dr. Eydie Miller, introduced her to Dr. Higginbotham. Dr. Ross said her biggest initial challenge was nervousness, given Dr. Higginbotham's stature in the field.

She provided an example of Dr. Higginbotham's sponsorship. When Dr. Ross sought research funding, Dr. Higginbotham stopped her in the middle of a busy clinic to suggest she apply for a Harold Amos Faculty Development Award (see Chapter 6 for more information on this program funded by the Robert Wood Johnson Foundation). Beyond the suggestion, however, Dr. Higginbotham introduced her to former recipients who explained the application process and expectations so that Dr. Ross could apply with greater focus and confidence. She added that when Dr. Ross received the fellowship (only the third ophthalmologist to do so in the history of the program), Dr. Higginbotham said it was one of the best feelings that she herself experienced in her career.

Dr. Higginbotham said time is a challenge in serving as a mentor or sponsor, but the need to increase minority representation in her field means she makes the time. She also noted the challenge in finding funding awards in surgical subspecialties. "When I learn about an opportunity in our field, I am proactive," Dr. Higginbotham said, adding that Dr. Ross "always follows up. That is critically important for the relationship." Dr. Ross agreed and emphasized, "Your mentor or your sponsor wants to see when they plant a seed, what sprouts from it. Staying in communication is important—it's a relationship." She also stressed that she prioritizes suggestions or requests she receives from her sponsor. "If Dr. Higginbotham asks me to do something, it is not 'let me see if I can find the time to do it.' It's 'when do you need it done?'" Dr. Ross said.

Dr. Ross added that, to her, they do not have a horizontal relationship but a vertical one. As Dr. Ross has progressed in her career and secured her lab, she said the relationship has changed, but acknowledged, "I still get nervous speaking with her. If I operate on one of her patients, I want the outcome to be perfect." She said she used to agonize over the emails she sent, carefully checking for spelling or grammatical mistakes, but realized that "I don't have time for long dissertation emails anymore. And I even text her!" She said she still has trouble calling Dr. Higginbotham by her first name, despite the latter's invitation to do so.

Dr. Higginbotham agreed with the importance of touching base and communications. She also shared characteristics of effective mentors and sponsors drawn from a paper by Diane Magrane and colleagues (see Table 4-1).

Speaking as both a mentee and now a mentor to medical students, Dr. Ross said, "A lesson learned is that communication and availability are important in mentoring relationships. I have standing meetings with my mentees. I want to see them progress. And if I can't help them do that, I want to get them to the next person who *can* help them progress." She noted sometimes a mentee will debate about possible options on topics that range from career decision to patient care. "As a mentor, it is exciting for a mentee to question me," she said. "It means they are actively thinking about the complexity of the topic. I also view it as an opportunity to grow myself."

TABLE 4-1 Characteristics of Effective Mentors and Sponsors

Characteristics of an Effective Mentor	Characteristics of an Effective Sponsor
Provide mentee/protégé with candid feedback	Publicly acknowledge their talents and achievements
Discuss strategies for managing interpersonal politics	Publicly support when they make a difficult or unpopular decision
Encourage attendance at internal or external leadership programs	Appoint to internal or external high-level committees/task forces
Seek feedback about how they are doing in new leadership positions	Directly nominate for advancement and prestigious positions
Set aside meetings on your calendar for regular mentoring	Assign them to an administrative role that tests new management skills, especially those with profit and loss responsibility
Advise them on executive presence and communication	Introduce them to individuals or groups to extend their professional networks
Guide them in development of an intentional and strategic plan for advance	Send in your place to important meetings, speaking appearances, and events
Provide opportunity for shadowing.	Provide opportunities to present to executive groups
	Pave the entry to leadership by preparing other faculty for the new leader's role
	Provide funding and resources for leadership program participation or coaching
	Engage team of advisors and consultants to advance the protégé
	Advocate with colleagues to advance the protégé

SOURCE: Eve Higginbotham, Workshop Presentation, December 7, 2020, from Magrane et al., 2018.

Gilda Barabino, Ph.D., and Shereka Banton, Ph.D.

Dr. Barabino recounted a time when she was a new professor at Georgia Tech in 2007, after 18 years at Northeastern University, and assigned to three problem-based sections. Dr. Banton stood out as one of the few Black students, of any gender, across the sections, and her quiet leadership and brilliance made her stand out even further in her group of students. Dr.

Barabino asked Dr. Banton whether she wanted to undertake undergraduate research in her lab. "As Dr. Dzirasa said, part of my motivation was to create a better version of myself," Dr. Barabino said.

Dr. Banton welcomed the connection with a Black woman professor. "I had the opportunity to show her what I could do and have a connection with someone I could view as a role model," she said. "I understood, even as an undergrad, how difficult it is for women and underrepresented minorities to rise to the leadership she had achieved in engineering." With Dr. Barabino's encouragement, Dr. Banton undertook research in sickle cell disease. Dr. Barabino pointed out she chose sickle cell as her career-long research because she could apply engineering principles to a medical problem, especially for a disease that disproportionately impacts African Americans and provides an opportunity to give back to the community. In addition, the research is at the intersection of politics, race, and health. Through the research, engineers participate in tying technical solutions with policy and social sciences. She shared these observations with Dr. Banton, who also pursued sickle cell research.

Dr. Banton said she became interested in both the science and the policy and public health implications of the research. She noted that Dr. Barabino's advocacy for her to be involved in areas that are atypical for most engineering students was critical and positioned her for success. Unusual for an engineering student, she interacted with patients and staff at the Medical College of Georgia and engaged in the public policy arena. Dr. Barabino supported her application for a fellowship with the Center for the Study of the Presidency and Congress. Universities send candidates from different departments to Washington, D.C., where they write papers about issues that the President and Congress can address. Dr. Banton's paper on health policy and underrepresented minorities received the program's most original paper award. She went on to an internship in the National Science Foundation's Directorate for Education and Human Resources focusing on the progression of underrepresented minorities in science and engineering. She said she was able to bring the perspective of someone living through the experience. "It was a huge opportunity for me to be able to offer that real-life experience, what it is like to be a Black woman in engineering," she said.

Dr. Barabino added:

> The mentor-mentee relationship is a two-way street. I learned as much from [Dr. Banton] as she has learned from me. In the paper and some of the work that she was doing at the National Science

> Foundation, one of the things she pointed out was the lack of progress despite interventions. I was on a committee looking at that issue and was able to use her report. There's much that is interchangeable and much we can learn from one another, which is so exciting.

When she accepted a new position in New York, Dr. Barabino said one of the hardest things was telling her mentees and advisees, Dr. Banton among them. "We talked about what the move would mean not just for my career but for the mentees and the people in my lab," she recalled. "I was so taken by her support of me and my career, when I was so worried about her career." Dr. Banton moved to New York to complete her research in Dr. Barabino's new lab, but the transition speaks to a larger issue of how these relationships adapt to change and upheaval, they both said.

Dr. Banton agreed with the characterization of mentorships as a two-way street. She recounted her reaction when Dr. Barabino announced she was leaving Georgia Tech. "I wanted to see her continue to blaze the trails that she was blazing," Dr. Banton said of her mentor. "One of the aspects of really successful mentoring relationships is that in addition to its being a situation where the mentee stands to benefit, the mentor can benefit as well." She explained she became invested in seeing Dr. Barabino's career progress, and looked to play whatever role she could as Dr. Barabino's student. She noted in academic circles, mentees and advisees represent their professor, and she sought to do this professionally.

Another role for mentors is to help mentees navigate external factors, said Dr. Barabino, and she helps her mentees with the socialization skills needed to succeed in the profession. She said she tries to be as transparent as possible about her own experiences in order to guide the experiences of Dr. Banton and others. Speaking of the external factors, Dr. Banton added, "One of the realities about the absence of Black people or any group is an assumption about the competence or the innate talent of that group. From the student perspective, it was important to have a role model to see that assumption is not true…. Having Dr. Barabino in my support system and network has been extremely helpful in countering outside perceptions."

DISCUSSION

The discussion began with a question about best practices in seeking a mentor. Dr. Dzirasa suggested identifying a potential mentor, then taking the initiative, even if means approaching the person multiple times. "Gently and jokingly, I would say to learn to stalk a good mentor," he said. That might mean finding yourself in the spaces where the person normally is and making the opportunity as easy as possible for the mentor. "In the long run, it is worth the time and effort," he said. Dr. Allsop and Dr. Banton also suggested making a personal connection and not just being transactional to secure a recommendation. Dr. Ross suggested having a clear expectation of "what you want from a mentor." She added, "Not every mentor or sponsor who helps you will be what you believe is nurturing. A lot of good mentors I've had are not interested in being my friend, they are interested in me achieving a certain goal." Dr. Dzirasa also suggested the importance to recognize the value of both the mentor's and the mentee's time. "Every good mentor knows how to write a grant, and you don't need 20 mentors to teach you to do the same thing 20 different ways." Instead, he suggested, "Be introspective to figure out what you need from a mentor."

In answer to a question from Ms. Yallowitz, Dr. Ross elaborated on why she considers Dr. Higginbotham a sponsor, rather than a mentor. "A mentor to me may be behind the scenes in terms of suggesting what I should do and might foster some relationships. A sponsor like Dr. Higginbotham has lobbied from her standing in the ophthalmology world on my behalf. She becomes my cheerleader, and she makes the connections." Dr. Barabino commented that while the same person can serve as a mentor or sponsor, "one distinction is that sponsors usually are in a position in their careers to advocate at a higher level." Dr. Dzirasa commented that he has sought people who can help him as both sponsors and mentors.

Discussion took place about the importance of having a mentor of the same gender, race, or other attributes. Based on his own experience, Dr. Allsop disagreed with the premise of a question by one attendee that strong personal relationships are more likely between women. Dr. Ross commented it is very rare to find one person who is a complete match; as she said, "That person does not exist, because that person is me!" For example, 4 years ago, she had her first child, and she is now experiencing a different career path than her mentor, a Black woman in her field who does not have children. Similarly, Dr. Allsop said he values the advice of his Ph.D. advisor, but they both recognized that she had a different path then he did. She "went out of her way to ensure the gaps were covered," he said, such as by connecting him with Dr. Dzirasa.

Dr. Banton suggested getting a sense of a potential mentor's vision to see whether there is a match of ideals and values. Sometimes, the panelists acknowledged, the relationship is not a good fit. "I have been on both sides," Dr. Dzirasa said. "As a mentor, I can ascertain how good a fit it is by how the mentee navigates my time and advice, and I have said to mentees that I think there may be someone else better aligned with their interests. From my end, trying to seek mentorship, I assume that maybe one out of five will pay off, but that is more than enough to shape my career. I try not to internalize failure." Regardless of how the mentor and mentee came together, Dr. Barabino said, "You may need to cut ties. Extended bad relationships do not work for anyone."

Dr. Reede closed the session by thanking the participants for sharing perspectives and their authenticity. "What is very clear is that each of you have formed long-term relationships built on trust and understanding."

REFERENCE

Magrane, D., P. S. Morahan, S. Ambrose, and S. Dannels. 2018. Competencies and practices in academic engineering leadership development: Lessons for a national survey. *Social Science* 7(10): 171. DOI:10.3390/socsci7100171.

5

Social Science—What Is Needed

Highlights from the Presentations

- Intersectionality is important to keep in mind in mentoring, coaching, and sponsorship, in which both parties have multiple identities related to race, gender, occupation, and much more (Dr. Blake-Beard).
- Protective hesitation and protective defensiveness can dampen giving and receiving authentic feedback, especially across dimensions of difference (Dr. Blake-Beard).
- Training is needed for both mentors and mentees; just having good intentions to mentor or be a mentee is less effective (Dr. Blake-Beard).
- To create a racially inclusive workplace, it is important to acknowledge how race shapes organizations, societies, and lives; affirm the value of racial diversity and the growth and potential for advancement for underrepresented minorities; and act to create a climate where racial diversity, justice, and inclusion can thrive (Dr. Morgan Roberts).
- While addressing all forms of discrimination is important, diversity efforts that are too broad mostly serve the people who are already in power (Dr. Morgan Roberts).

- Strategically managing one's career and brand are necessary to advance; it is not enough to assume one's work will speak for itself (Dr. Morgan Roberts).

Mentoring, coaching, and sponsorship occur in a variety of settings and transition points. Orlando Kirton, M.D., M.B.A., Abington-Jefferson Health, moderated a panel in which two social scientists discussed these relationships and the environments in which they play out. Stacy Blake-Beard, Ph.D., Dartmouth University and Simmons College, focused on mentoring, coaching, and sponsorship as sources of critical support and feedback. Laura Morgan Roberts, Ph.D., University of Virginia, spoke about racially just workplaces to advance true inclusion of people with diverse talents. A robust question-and-answer period followed their presentations.

SOURCES OF CRITICAL SUPPORT AND FEEDBACK

Dr. Blake-Beard said she would build on the insights brought out by the previous panel of mentors and mentees. She noted mentoring, coaching, and sponsorship relationships are important to her both as a course of study over the past decades and in her own development.

Referring to the earlier discussion about mentoring across races, genders, and other characteristics, she identified the concept of intersectionality (Crenshaw, 1989) as the recognition that people have different identities, and they learn from each other based on both similarities and differences. "To give a name to what others have brought up, when we show up, we show up as more than one thing with many dimensions of our identities. There are challenges and opportunities when we acknowledge this," she said.

Although the concepts intermingle and play off each other, she defined the different relationships:

> Mentoring is a dynamic, reciprocal relationship with a caring individual, a sharing of experience of wisdom, and a readiness and willingness to enrich the professional development of both people.... Sponsorship is action oriented and is focused on positioning and on helping the person receiving the sponsorship move ahead. The sponsors are available, willing, and even eager to use their networks to help with the advancement of their colleague, publicly

and behind closed doors. Coaching is more focused on a particular competency or skill, with a need met around a specific goal.

Benefits gained from a mentor include hearing clear and realistic expectations, active listening and thinking about how to help, and self-disclosure and thus vulnerability. It is necessary to be willing to take risks and be proactive in getting a mentor. Managing feedback from the mentor or sponsor is often not explicitly discussed, but it is important to learn how to use that feedback, she added.

There are challenges, especially for people of color, in getting support. She noted none of these ideas will seem new to participants, but it is important to give names to them and consider how they are interrelated. They include tokenism, "that aspect of our lives where we stand out because we are one of few." A dilemma is how to get close to another person and share thoughts and feelings without being perceived as too close. Stereotypes exist; she referred participants to the implicit association test[1] that can help reveal a person's implicit biases and internal stereotypes and how quickly inferences are made.

How to get real feedback from a mentor, not just general positive reinforcement, is also a challenge, especially when the relationship occurs across dimensions of difference (e.g., race, gender, institutional type). Particularly related to race and ethnicity, she pointed to the concepts of protective hesitation and protective defensiveness. In protective hesitation, "the mentor doesn't give honest feedback out of fear of being perceived as racist, homophobic, sexist, or any other dimension." Yet, she noted, this can result in not offering feedback that the mentee should have. Dr. Blake-Beard considered this as "protecting myself [as the mentor], not the mentee. The irony is in trying not to hurt the recipient, the mentee *is* hurt because they do not get full information." Protective defensiveness can also occur, in which people of color build a shell around themselves in situations where they stand out as a minority. "The challenge is what if that shell gets so thick, feedback that you need will not penetrate it. The irony is that in trying to protect ourselves so much, we do not hear what we need, such as how to apply for a position."

Accessing support means paying attention to whom to ask for support, when to ask, and how to ask. "You may have to figure out a way to connect with them," she pointed out. "All these people at the heart of it want you

---

[1] See https://www.projectimplicit.net.

to succeed. But to provide that support, there has to be a two-way street." She suggested keeping intersectionality in mind, and overcoming both protective hesitation and protective defensiveness.

She also stressed the need not to have just one relationship to draw on for support, but to have a network that includes peers, friends and family, advisors, and professional associations. She noted a saying, "If you want to go fast, go alone; if you want to go far, go with others."

TOWARD A RACIALLY JUST WORKPLACE

Dr. Morgan Roberts said she was asked to place the workshop conversations in the context of organizational change, and specifically how mentoring, coaching, and sponsoring fit within a broader suite of initiatives with respect to leading racially just organizations. She drew from two edited volumes she published on the topic (Roberts et al., 2016; Roberts et al., 2019), with more than 50 studies from more than 100 global scholars about what it means to truly value difference in organizations. Three interrelated steps are critical: acknowledging, affirming, and acting. She noted her more recent book, *Race, Work, and Leadership*, includes a contribution by Dr. Blake-Beard.

The social science perspective is useful because of the interrelatedness between the economic, education, housing, justice, and health sectors, she said. In 2020, the Business Roundtable, whose members are CEOs from leading corporations, committed to advancing racial justice across these sectors in recognition that the issues have implications for the viability of the economy (Business Roundtable, 2020). Long-standing and perpetual problems related to wealth inequality and income disparities have been exacerbated by the COVID-19 pandemic. The wage gap as a function of inequality and racism has largely remained unchanged for decades, and the numbers are even more sobering because of the pandemic. When talking about diversity broadly stated, she pointed out that some of the nuances are lost, because the experiences of Black professionals are different from those of people of Latinx and Asian origin.

Black people comprise about 3 percent of senior executive positions, about the same as in health-care leadership. There seems to be a ceiling, even though diversity is stated as a goal for society and the economy. "Diversity of thought jolts us into cognitive action in a way that homogeneity does not," she said, referring to work by Katherine Phillips (2014). "But the lived experience fails to deliver on that promise." She has focused her recent writing on the disconnect in many organizations between the promise of hiring a diverse or more culturally competent workforce and doing the work to value differences. This, she said, is where relational work like mentoring, coaching, and sponsoring comes in.

Even if diversity is a stated goal based on business needs, most do not want to "put in the work and make the investment to build the relationships," she said. Protective hesitation and defensiveness, as explained earlier by Dr. Blake-Beard, come into play. Despite underinvestment in building a diverse workforce, there is an expectation to receive returns. There is also a moral case for doing the right thing, stemming from what has been inflicted on Black and Brown people, often by medical institutions, including in enslavement and post-enslavement. Specifically,

> If we as institutions truly want to move forward and make mentoring, coaching, and sponsorship more than a voluntary one-off exchange but really baked into the system, we need to keep top of mind the moral case as well as the business case for doing so.

Empirical research that she has undertaken identifies challenges that Black and Brown professionals face in health care, higher education, financial services, nonprofits, and other fields. She and colleagues identified common patterns across sectors, which she categorized as the "Four A's": access (increasing representation in the pipeline); authenticity (building inclusion and belonging); advancement (getting ahead); and authority and accountability (having to struggle for respect as Black professionals). In research she and Dr. Blake-Beard did in the Boston area, they learned many Black health-care professionals were recruited into clinical care positions to meet underserved communities but overlooked when it was time to pick new leaders. Many left Boston or health care entirely because they felt they could not advance in the system.

As the daughter and sister of physicians, Dr. Morgan Roberts said she has listened to them and other Black doctors talk about repeated experiences with microaggressions. They speak of being mistaken as someone without a medical degree and treated with less respect. They often receive career advice that indicates lowered expectations or pigeon-holing into certain roles. "These dynamics undermine authority, and the systems are not held accountable," she said. Black physicians and other health-care professionals are carrying the burden of a cognitive or emotional tax, and feel less connected. The promise of diversity that will bring resources to benefit patients and society becomes undermined. Professionals of color cannot bring their full authentic selves or identities to the workplace, and instead tuck themselves behind a protective mask.

She noted the concern about violence and oppression expressed during the summer of 2020. Institutions pledged to make changes in the service of greater freedom and equality. But what happens in institutions is a pivot from designing intentional programs for high-performing Black professionals to what she termed "what about-isms"—that is, what about other marginalized groups. She stressed that she did not disagree with this concern, but broadening the aperture can shift attention away from addressing violence and oppression against Black people. "Over time, we include everything, and therefore do not address much of anything except the comfort level of the people who are most powerful," she observed.

Dr. Morgan Roberts returned to the three areas of acknowledging, affirming, and acting to engage people's heads, hearts, and hands. It involves, she said, acknowledging how race shapes organizations, societies, and lives; affirming the value of racial diversity and the growth and potential for advancement for underrepresented minorities; and acting to create a climate where racial diversity, justice, and inclusion can thrive. That climate, she added, will benefit everyone. She invited leaders to take up this affirmation: "Acknowledging the presence of bias and affirming the value of difference will not diminish the worth of my contributions or the validity of my hardships."

Dr. Morgan Roberts urged caution with "one size fits all" related to diversity, since it tends to move people back into their comfort zones and not address the needs of the most vulnerable. Creating cultures of inquiry around race is important, but people often avoid conversation about race. Individuals must remain open to learning; interested in having conversations about race; curious about organization's practices; willing to use data-based decision-making about admissions, promotions, and funding; and prepared to call out subtle and overt discrimination. "Invite people to tell their stories," she urged. "What does race mean to you? What is your 'why' for engaging in this work?"

She shared her own "why" for her engagement by closing with several photographs that included a new memorial to enslaved laborers at the University of Virginia (UVA), in front of which members of the UVA Health system knelt in honor of George Floyd. She noted her own connections with UVA, as a current faculty member, alumna, and descendant of family members on her mother's side who worked as cooks at the university in the 1800s.

DISCUSSION

Dr. Kirton asked Dr. Blake-Beard about the role of coaches. She said career development is a "team sport," and people need different supports at different times in their careers, as the previous panel highlighted. The two presenters commented on the fact that they have "created a team for each other." When Dr. Morgan Roberts was an undergraduate at UVA considering a Ph.D. in psychology, her advisor was an alumnus of the University of Michigan, as was Dr. Blake-Beard. "I cold-called her," Dr. Morgan Roberts recounted. Dr. Blake-Beard helped guide her as she applied to graduate school and entered the job market. Over the years, they have had a "multiplex" set of relationships. Dr. Blake-Beard echoed previous comments by stressing that the relationship goes both ways.

A participant asked how to approach unconscious bias and microaggressions. Dr. Morgan Roberts replied that it depends on "your frame of reference and sphere of influence." As a bystander, she drew on the saying, "If you see something, say something. One of the simplest things is to be on alert and vigilant about stereotypical comments, even in the form of a joke or teasing." But she noted situations, such as going on rounds as a medical student and hearing a disparaging comment about a patient, when the student does not have the power to say anything. "I get that. But if you do have more power, speak up." As a direct target rather than a bystander, she recommends "picking your battles." She noted she wrote articles for *Harvard Business Review* with tips, including to "pause, call attention, and inquire" (Roberts and Washington, 2020; Roberts et al., 2020).

Offering to serve as a mentor, especially across races and genders, was also discussed when a participant asked for recommendations about how to reach out to more junior faculty with an offer to mentor. "Let people know you are available by your activities and how you send out messages," Dr. Blake-Beard suggested. "People will not naturally assume you are willing. Be thoughtful—be explicit that you want to support people across the dimensions of difference and offer opportunities that get over the natural walls and boundaries that people put up." With Dr. Audrey Murrell, she edited a book on this topic (Murrell and Blake-Beard, 2017) that includes a chapter co-authored by Dr. Morgan Roberts, as well as a chapter co-authored by Dr. Barabino and Dr. Banton (see Chapter 4). When she started her graduate career in 1989, "people didn't talk about mentoring across differences. Mentoring was about white men mentoring other white men." She also noted the concepts apply internationally.

The presenters were asked about differences in mentoring Ph.D. versus medical graduates for career success. Dr. Morgan Roberts said, "With mentoring and medical graduates, there is a tension whether you are pursuing a career in academic medicine or one that is primarily or exclusively clinical." Some elements may draw more Black medical graduate students into clinical practice, including financial needs and incentives. Her dissertation and a follow-up survey focused on Black medical students and the tensions they feel in definitions of success, especially when they are shouldering high levels of student debt. Mentors may struggle with helping students understand how they can pursue various paths and still feel they are contributing to the community, she commented. She pointed out the parallels in Ph.D. training, and in choosing between a tenure-track career at an R1 institution or work in the world of practice. "These are some of the complexities that may create more similarities for [doctoral and medical school] Black students who are trying to figure out how to pursue success on their terms."

Dr. Blake-Beard elaborated on mentoring across dimensions of differences. The mentoring literature talks about mentoring across phases and stages. A relationship starts with an initiation phase of how to connect with each other, be vulnerable, and share. Subsequent stages cover cultivation of the relationship, possibly followed by separation in which the two people move apart and must decide whether they want to recommit. Mentoring across differences is not easy, and there will be times when the two people move apart from one another, and they may or may not come back together.

In terms of making the business case for organizational change, Dr. Morgan Roberts listed three outcomes of interest: intellectual capital (growing and developing a set of cognitive resources to solve problems); organizational effectiveness (to improve efficiency and benefit from the contributions and questions of people usually on the margins); and innovation (diversity of thought to tackle systems-level challenges). To these three, she added the business case needs to account for sustainability. "How are we continuing to grow and develop a diverse and representative set of leaders who will help us operate to build a stronger society?" Sustainability is often related to climate change and the environment. In health care, sustainability relates to wage inequality, as greater than 70 percent of lowest-wage workers in health-care systems are women of color and are exposed to all forms of toxicity. "If our business case for diversity is only about having more people at the top and then we declare victory, that is short sighted," she said, and pointed to ground-breaking research by Adia Harvey Wingfield (2019) about the unique experiences and hardships across class in health-care settings. "To bring together moral and desirable business outcomes in making the business case, we must think of the whole system," she said. Dr. Blake-Beard noted that organizational research in which she has been involved also takes into consideration what happens if diversity is *not* addressed, such as retention and reputation.

Dr. Reede asked about issues related to Black people advancing to leadership positions in organizations. Dr. Morgan Roberts said the Boston study identified as a barrier the lack of socialization into leadership and administration. Gifted medical care providers are not automatically skilled managers or administrators. Given the professional underrepresentation of Black adults in managerial and administrative roles, most Black medical students and graduates did not grow up in this world. They feel they are "late to the party" to acquire the informal socialization needed to succeed in leadership roles. Many try to compensate in positive ways by pursuing higher education. Another study that looked at 50 years of Black graduates from Harvard Business School (HBS) found they were more likely than white graduates to have more pedigrees from a resume standpoint, such as having graduated from higher-ranked institutions before matriculating at HBS or earning joint degrees while getting their M.B.A.s. Another dynamic was many respondents said they were actively discouraged at various points from pursuing leadership roles.

A participant asked for advice for newly hired Black faculty who find they are forced to operate at a lower level than they had expected. Dr. Morgan Roberts suggested "strategically managing visibility.... When we feel overwhelmed and defensive, we adopt a strategy that undermines our advancement, in which we say we are going to put our heads down and let the work speak for itself." Instead, she said it is important to be proactive in networking relationships, be transparent, and frame one's strengths and contributions in terms of leadership. Dr. Blake-Beard added that this situation speaks to intersectionality. Having individual agency does not erase the problems of structural racism, but given the challenges of structural racism, it is important to navigate and strengthen one's agency. Dr. Morgan Roberts added that allyship has been another recently discussed concept, and sometimes it is important to find the right allies who can do diversity work because of their privilege. Confidantes are needed who can provide authentic feedback, said Dr. Kirton. Dr. Morgan Roberts agreed. Twenty years ago, when they both lived in Boston, she and Dr. Blake-Beard often met for dinner to support each other. As "one of the only," the spotlight is bright, she observed.

When asked about a mentor training framework, Dr. Blake-Beard suggested several effective practices. It takes more than just commitment. Both mentors and mentees need training and support, beginning with a solid orientation. Dr. Morgan Roberts said she has seen "an ebb and flow" in institutional practices. The University of Michigan set explicit diversity targets and held itself accountable for achieving those targets, and the university was sued. Research findings from the 1990s seemed to be gaining traction, but an adverse response also occurred, she said, as shown by the fact there are fewer Black men in medical education now than 30 years ago.

Steps to reinvigorate initiatives go back to what has been shown to work, Dr. Morgan Roberts said. These steps include buying into the value of diversity, not equivocating, looking holistically at the characteristics that people bring to a situation, and defining leadership competencies through the lens of inclusion. Corporations are setting financial targets around hiring and promotion, she added. The Nasdaq just announced that companies that want to be listed on their exchange must disclose the racial and gender composition of their boards and have at least two diverse candidates within 4 years. There is still work to do, she said, but the bottom line is companies are starting to be more explicit about setting expectations, tying to CEO compensation, credentialing, and rewarding individuals.

In response to a question from Dr. Morgan Roberts about what she is hopeful about, Dr. Blake-Beard said she is hopeful that people realize that the future depends on raising and making visible these issues. Dr. Morgan Roberts said she is hopeful that people are talking about these issues more openly and publicly than even a few years ago. Dr. Kirton suggested the brutality around George Floyd's death and the COVID-19 pandemic may present a generational opportunity for transformative change. Dr. Blake-Beard said the benefits to diversity are global, although Dr. Morgan Roberts warned there must also be a level-set of expectations: "Representation is one piece and there has been progress, but it is a journey and we must remain committed."

The workshop co-chairs closed the session and the first day of the workshop. Dr. Morgan Roberts thanked the participants for providing a unique experience and provocative thinking. Knowledge from different directions provides clues about how to improve hospitals, medical schools, and other organizations. Dr. Reede stressed the need to keep in mind the arc of careers beyond medical school to different points of transition. Racism at societal, institutional, and individual levels can hinder achievement, she said, and she thanked participants for their clarity and commitment in blazing trails and preparing others to continue the work. She said conversations such as those that have taken place at this workshop need to be part of the conversation in the academy, academic medical centers, research organizations, government, and in public and private spaces.

REFERENCES

Business Roundtable. 2020. Business Roundtable CEOs Announce Corporate Actions, Public Policy Recommendations to Advance Racial Equity and Justice, Increase Economic Opportunities in America. https://www.businessroundtable.org/business-roundtable-ceos-announce-corporate-actions-public-policy-recommendations-to-advance-racial-equity-and-justice-increase-economic-opportunity-in-america.

Crenshaw, K. 1989. Demarginalizing the intersection of race and sex: A Black feminist critique of antidiscrimination doctrine, feminist theory, and antiracist politics. *University of Chicago Legal Forum* 1989(8). https://chicagounbound.uchicago.edu/uclf/vol1989/iss1/8/.

Murrell, A., and S. Blake-Beard (eds.). 2017. *Mentoring Diverse Leaders: Creating Change for People, Processes, and Paradigms.* New York: Taylor & Francis.

Phillips, K. 2014. How diversity makes us smarter. *Scientific American*. https://www.scientificamerican.com/article/how-diversity-makes-us-smarter/.

Roberts, L. M., A. J. Mayo, and D. A. Thomas (eds.). 2019. *Race, Work, and Leadership: New Perspectives on the Black Experience*. Cambridge, MA: Harvard Business Press.

Roberts, L. M., C. L. McCluney, E. L. Thomas, and M. Kim. 2020. How U.S. companies can support employees of color through the pandemic. *Harvard Business Review* (May 22).

Roberts, L. M., and E. Washington. 2020. U.S. businesses must take meaningful action against racism. *Harvard Business Review*. https://hbr.org/2020/06/u-s-businesses-must-take-meaningful-action-against-racism.

Roberts, L. M., L. P. Wooten, and M. N. Davidson (eds.). 2016. *Positive Organizing in a Just Society: Understanding and Engaging Differences for Capacity Building and Inclusion*. New York: Taylor and Routledge.

Wingfield, A. H. 2019. *Flatlining: Race, Work, and Health Care in the New Economy.* Berkeley: University of California Press.

6

Program Models and Best Practices

Highlights from the Presentations

- The commitment of a long-serving, illustrious National Advisory Council is a driving force behind the Harold Amos Program because its members select scholars, serve as mentors, evaluate progress, perform site visits, and intervene when necessary (Ms. Ardery).
- Building community within a cohort is key to scalability (Ms. Ardery).
- A virtual community that provides peer and expert coaching can improve the academic productivity of minority early-stage investigators (Dr. Ofili).
- An Individual Development Plan provides a way to set, account for, and revise professional goals (Dr. Ofili).
- Leaders of color need to develop social and organizational competencies related to acumen, attitude, and aptitude (Dr. Reede).
- The continued engagement by alumni of fellowship and other programs strengthens their leadership capacities and opportunities (Dr. Reede).
- Rather than a pipeline, a highway with "on" and "off" ramps may serve as a more useful model for physician-scientist training (Dr. Ajijola).

- Data show the direct and indirect benefits to an institution by investing in flexible physician-scientist programs (Dr. Ajijola).

Valerae Lewis, M.D., University of Texas MD Anderson Cancer Center, moderated a session to learn from representatives of five programs. Nina Ardery, M.A., M.B.A., Harold Amos Medical Faculty Development Program, launched the session. She was followed by Elizabeth Ofili, M.D., M.P.H., F.A.C.C., Morehouse School of Medicine (MSM); Joan Reede, M.D., M.P.H., M.S., M.B.A., Harvard Medical School; and Olujimi Ajijola, M.D., Ph.D., University of California, Los Angeles (UCLA). Each gave a history of the program in which they are involved, best practices, outcomes and lessons for upscaling it, and outlook for the future.

HAROLD AMOS MEDICAL FACULTY DEVELOPMENT PROGRAM

Ms. Ardery described the Harold Amos Program supported by the Robert Wood Johnson Foundation. It began with a proposal from the foundation staff to the board in 1983 that recommended "the Foundation initiate a new program to increase the number of minority medical faculty with high likelihood of achieving senior academic positions in the nation's medical schools." It is a 4-year mentored research training program in which, Ms. Ardery emphasized, "we fund people, not projects; we are looking for people who will become leaders." About 100 people from underrepresented backgrounds apply each year, and they provide information about their mentors as part of their written applications. About 25 finalists are interviewed; even reaching this stage is an accomplishment, she said, recognizing the process can be nerve-wracking for applicants. She acknowledged previous recipients, including Dr. Lewis and Dr. Ahmara Ross (see Chapter 4).

The 39th cohort will be selected in summer 2021 in medicine, dentistry, and nursing. The program began with basic biomedical research but has expanded to include clinical investigation and health services research and epidemiology. The foundation funds 10 fellows each year, with additional awards funded by three partners (American Society of Hematology, American Society of Nephrology, and American Heart Association). The partner-funded scholars are part of each year's cohort.

Strengths of the program are the strong commitment by and composition of the National Advisory Committee (NAC); well-vetted mentors;

"360 mentorship" (fellows apply with a mentor, are assigned a mentor, have the cohort as a network, and serve as mentors themselves); an annual meeting to provide scientific and leadership training; and interdisciplinary exposure. Additional strengths include the longevity of the staff and the NAC; professional and personal networking; and a highly supportive family atmosphere and environment. The three partnerships mentioned above provide benefits in the form of additional funding for scholars and sources for speakers, memberships, and conference participation, among other benefits.

The commitment of the NAC is the driving force of the program, Ms. Ardery said. Its members select the scholars, serve as mentors, evaluate progress, perform site visits, and intervene when necessary. Nine alumni are now on the NAC. Among the outcomes (see Box 6-1), greater than 80 percent of the scholars remain in academic medicine. A recent study compared interviewees who did and did not get the award. There were small differences in their academic ranks and publications, but the real differences were in the leadership roles that the alumni went on to assume, Ms. Ardery said.

Scalability is helped by the partnerships that allow for a larger program. Building community also aids scalability, she stressed, because scholars do

BOX 6-1
Harold Amos Program Results

Of the approximately 325 alumni as of October 2020:

- Greater than 80 percent have remained in academic medicine
- 8 deans or presidents
- 103 full professors
- 81 associate professors
- 62 assistant professors
- 2 current and 1 former National Institutes of Health director
- 18 in private practice, 13 in industry (in research)
- Several presidents of societies
- 2 state secretaries of health
- 1 MacArthur "genius grant" recipient, astronaut, and person whose life story was optioned by Brad Pitt

SOURCE: Nina Ardery, Workshop Presentation, December 8, 2020.

not want to disappoint members of their cohort. Related to mentorship, she noted that the NAC mentors are not necessarily in the field of the scholars, but they provide a helpful outside voice. An alumni group also provides support. They help scholars prioritize their time and capabilities. "Mentors need to be allies in helping scholars focus on the work that can lead to their advancement and need to learn to be able to say no," she commented. "The scholars are not diversity experts, and many find themselves being asked to do things they are not trained to do."

Ms. Ardery highlighted a few changes in the program over time. It began just for physicians but has now expanded to nurses and dentists. The definition of minority has expanded to Latinx, African American, Native American, and other members of historically disadvantaged groups. The partnerships are also relatively new, and the program places more emphasis on the cohorts to intentionally build peer groups. A leadership academy has also been added. In terms of those not selected, Ms. Ardery said all are competitive applicants and if the program had more funding, it would expand.

VIRTUAL COMMUNITY TO SUPPORT DIVERSE EARLY-STAGE INVESTIGATORS

Dr. Ofili spoke about a collaboration between Morehouse School of Medicine, the W. Montague Cobb/National Medical Association (NMA) Health Institute, and the Association for Academic Minority Physicians (AAMP). It builds on the National Research Mentoring Network (NRMN), which was formed by the National Institutes of Health (NIH) to address lack of success primarily by African Americans in securing R01 funding. The program at MSM included coaching in grant writing and other supports, such as a Collaboratory that consists of a Slack platform to engage investigators with each other and with coaches. A recent article published in *PLOS One* details the results across NRMN and found the 22 percent success rate exceeded the 2016–2018 success rate for new R01s (Weber-Main et al., 2020).

In the second phase of NRMN, the Strategic Empowerment Tailored for Health Equity Investigators Model focused on the institutional climate and the ability of scholars to access sponsors. A randomized trial is testing the hypothesis that early-stage investigators (ESIs) who receive developmental network coaching through the Health Equity Collaboratory during a Grant Coaching Program (GCP) will have higher submission rates 6-month post-intervention than control group participants who participate in a GCP alone.

The Cobb/NMA Health Institute already had a program to recruit ESI.[1] The three organizations combined forces to provide more structure by forming a virtual community through the Collaboratory developed at MSM. Each Cobb Scholar develops an Individual Development Plan (IDP) and conducts a personal SWOT (strengths, weaknesses, opportunities, threats) analysis. Another aspect is access to mentors through AAMP, NRMN, and other networks. With these various components, Dr. Ofili explained, "We developed an adaptive approach. We could meet people where they are and help direct them to access other resources to be successful."

The model has received support from NIH. The target population is biomedical scientists, including M.D.s, health professions doctorates, and Ph.D. scientists, who are underrepresented in biomedical research, with women prioritized. Enrollment of postdoctoral scholars and junior faculty has begun. Following a rigorous interview process, 25 to 30 ESIs will be supported for 12 months. After a workshop at an AAMP meeting, they will participate in the Collaboratory and other activities. Each applicant will draft an IDP, adapted from the Indiana University Clinical and Translational Sciences Institute, and continue to refine their goals and analyses through the plan (see Box 6-2). The project also includes a resiliency survey, based on research about the relationship between resilience and academic productivity of minority faculty members (Cora-Bramble et al., 2010). Dr. Ofili noted the need to refine some of the materials based on lessons learned during the COVID-19 pandemic.

Cobb/NMA, AAMP, and MSM scholars have access to the *Journal of Racial and Ethnic Health Disparities*, networking and coaching support through the NRMN, access to clinical trials GCP training, and participation as site principal investigators. Outcomes looked at will include grant submissions to NIH and foundations, scholarly presentations at national meetings, and peer-reviewed publications. Other outcomes will include access to mentors and other resources, as well as individual and focus group evaluations of scholars' and mentors' experiences.

[1] For more information, see https://www.thecobbinstitute.org/overview.

BOX 6-2
Components of an Individual Career Development Plan

The National Medical Association/Cobb/Association for Academic Minority Physicians/Morehouse School of Medicine Scholars use an Individual Development Plan (IDP) as a tool to develop, plan, and empower their academic career. It consists of the following elements:

- Your values, passion, and vision
- SWOT (strengths, weaknesses, opportunities, threats) analysis: Your strengths and weaknesses
- Your professional goals
- Alignment of goals with departmental and school needs
- Time allocation
- Last year's success and challenges
- Assessing the viability of your IDP: Is it SMART? (Specific, Measurable, Attainable, Results oriented, Time limited or Time bound)
- Personal goals and work-life integration

SOURCE: Elizabeth Ofili, Workshop Presentation, December 8, 2020.

COMMONWEALTH FUND FELLOWSHIP IN MINORITY HEALTH POLICY AT HARVARD UNIVERSITY

Dr. Reede recalled conversations at Harvard in the 1990s that recognized the need to involve more minorities in policy making and leadership positions to narrow health disparities. When she was approached about designing a solution, she found the prevailing assumptions included a lack of minority professionals from whom to draw, as well as presumed lack of interest and preparedness. Potential and paths to leadership were seen through the limited lens of what traditionally had occurred, rather than more holistically or in new ways.

The Commonwealth Fund Fellowship at Harvard University (CFFHU) that emerged is a 1-year program with three major goals: (1) prepare physicians, particularly from groups underrepresented in medicine, to become leaders who improve the health of disadvantaged and vulnerable populations through transforming health-care delivery systems and promoting innovation in policies, practices, and programs that address health equity and the social determinants of health; (2) increase the representation of well-trained, creative minority physicians who are leaders in health, health-care delivery, government, foundation, private, and academic sectors; and (3) support the continued career development and advancement of alumni fellows in ways that enhance existing and create new resources that improve the communication, function, utilization, and meaningful actions of the alumni network.

One aspect of the program is course work to teach technical and cognitive skills that result in a degree in health policy or health management. Interpersonal, conceptual, and strategic skills are also imparted to assist people with entering leadership positions, starting in a more limited domain but expanding over time to become senior-level leaders in systems. A special focus is on developing social and organizational competencies relevant to leaders of color, including those related to cultural knowledge and awareness, communication, and leadership branding and aspirations, among others (Sy et al., 2017; see Table 6-1).

Program elements include leadership seminars and forums, a skills development series, shadowing, and a practicum. These elements provide role models, make pathways transparent and accessible, provide real work exposure, and examine the written and unwritten rules of success in action. A "mentor posse" is developed so that each fellow has multiple mentors such as alumni, faculty, the CFFHU advisory committee and administrators, underrepresented minority leaders, health system leaders, and discipline leaders. Considerations in identifying the mentors include the mentee's career goals, discipline/area of study, shared interests, shared values and commitment, capacity to expand the mentee's networks and provide sponsorship, and willingness to coach.

As fellows move forward after the first year, they continue to expand their networks, resources, and influence through an annual meeting for fellows and alumni to come together, site visits, and an alumni association (now its own 501c3 organization). These offerings provide continued leadership and skill development, decrease isolation, increase visibility, and offer opportunities for collaboration.

All 142 fellows to date remain engaged in policy, research, and/or service delivery related to minority health and vulnerable populations, Dr. Reede said. Close to 80 percent have academic appointments, and almost all serve on advisory committees and boards. Greater than 70 percent have had research published in peer-reviewed journals, and two-thirds have

TABLE 6-1 Social and Organizational Competencies Imparted through the Commonwealth Fund Fellowship in Minority Health Policy at Harvard University

Criteria	Social Competencies	Organizational Competencies
Acumen	Cultural Knowledge and Awareness • Mainstream culture • Own culture • Other marginalized culture • Professional culture	Rules of Success • Accessing written rules – within and across disciplines and organizational settings • Navigating the system - awareness and access to unwritten rules
	Communication • Cultural communication norms • Perceptions of accents, appearance, style • Oral and written presentation	Positioning • Identifying and utilizing mentors, coaches and sponsors • Using the Strategic "yes" and "no"
Aptitude	Social Decorum • Understanding social norms • Managing emotions • Managing response to microaggressions, bias and stereotypes • Building and managing professional networks	Leadership Branding • Managing visibility • Branding oneself • Promoting oneself • Asserting oneself
Attitude	Cultural Inclusion • Cultural identity • Cultural esteem • Cultural efficacy	Career Determinism • Owning ones career path • Managing career transitions • Pursuing employment and security
	Self construal and Evaluation • Self esteem • Self efficacy • Stereotype threat • Imposter syndrome	Leadership Aspiration • Recognizing biased perceptions of others re: leaders of color • Expanding leadership aspirations and awareness of options

SOURCE: Adapted from Joan Reede, Workshop Presentation, December 8, 2020. Revised from T. Sy et al., *Asian American Journal of Psychology*, 2017.

discussed public health and minority health issues in the popular media. Fellows continue to advance in their career trajectories and reach out to help one another. "This points to the need to build communities within communities. They come into the program as a cohort but they cross cohorts through the alumni association and other means." In conclusion, Dr. Reede said that CFFHU clearly shows there are minority individuals who have the potential, desire, and talents to move into leadership positions to create change. The issue is how to identify, nurture, and support them not just at one point in time, but also as they move forward across their careers.

In a short discussion that followed Dr. Reede's presentation, Dr. Lewis asked about efforts to mentor high school students. Dr. Reede said CFFHU fellows and others at Harvard are involved in a separate nonprofit that is also run out of her office, called the Biomedical Science Careers Program. It has matched 14,000 students at different levels with 1,500 volunteers.

Looking ahead, Dr. Reede said the need for leadership opportunities continues. She noted when CFFHU began, it was believed it might need to run 5 or 10 years. "People thought, won't that be enough? The answer is no. Many of us are at a point in our careers where we are asking who is going to replace us. We need more leaders across multiple disciplines and in multiple sectors. We have barely touched the tip of the iceberg to create the leaders of tomorrow."

Dr. Reede and the previous two presenters were asked how junior faculty can develop their own roadmaps to leadership. Dr. Ofili stressed flexibility. "Everyone can find a way to connect within their own environment to acquire the skills needed. Structured programs are important, but we also need programs that allow people the flexibility, as life goes on, to incorporate these efforts into their own growth and development." Dr. Reede pointed to the need for academic centers and other institutions to understand the importance of leadership and leadership development for their own best interests. Certificates, programs, sponsorships, fellowships, and other opportunities benefit the individuals and the organizations. Ms. Ardery added that institutions must value mentoring and consider it in tenure and promotions.

UCLA STAR PROGRAM

Dr. Ajijola reframed the so-named science, technology, engineering, and mathematics (STEM) pipeline as a set of highways with on-ramps and off-ramps for physician-scientist training. Although they are a small number overall, physician-scientists represent an outsized share of health leaders in academia, industry, and government. Yet, while Hispanic, Black, and Native Americans are about 30 percent of the population, the three groups together represented about 10 percent of M.D./Ph.D. matriculates in 2018–2019 and only 5 percent of NIH-funded physician-scientist investigators. The outlook for the future remains poor, he added.

The predominant training model in the United States is the Medical Scientist Training Program, which intersperses M.D. and Ph.D. clinical and research training over more than a decade. Before entry, in addition to academic excellence, applicants need to have conducted substantial research (in high school and increasingly in middle school, according to Dr. Ajijola), amass letters of recommendation, understand research careers, and be able to commit to an extended career path. Underrepresented minorities face barriers before entering this pipeline and as they move within it, as discussed throughout the workshop. Attrition along the pipeline means talent is lost at various stages, especially for underrepresented minorities. Dr. Ajijola countered that this pipeline is not the best way to envision diversifying the scientific workforce for two reasons:

> Pipeline models are problematic because they (1) nudge us to consider talent lost to attrition as unrecoverable and (2) do not nurture physician-scientist reentry into scientific training of the workforce.

The UCLA Specialty Training and Advanced Research (STAR) Program was set up in 1995 to rethink the pipeline metaphor by offering more flexible pathways, Dr. Ajijola said. Founded in 1995 by Linda Demer, M.D., Ph.D., and Alan Fogelman, M.D., it is designed for physicians interested in an investigative research career, allowing coordination of clinical specialty training with an advanced research program leading to a graduate degree. What is unique, he said, is that clinical and research training are integrated, at a ratio of 75 percent research and 25 percent clinical after the first year. Best practices include a unique individualized curriculum design for each trainee, an instructor-scale salary, and mentorship/sponsorship and networking across the campus. Also important, the department of medicine commits to support the trainees for the length of their research, and some of the trainees become clinical instructors when they are board-eligible. Other resources, such as grant-writing support and a community of trainees, are also available. Trainees can access all departments at UCLA, as well as the

California Institute of Technology and Pardee RAND Graduate School, to learn new methodologies.

The 25-year outcomes showed that 80 percent have remained in research, and about half have obtained an NIH or other career development award; 19 percent received an NIH R01 or equivalent grant or landed a leadership position in a STEM industry or other organization (Wong et al., 2016). NIH adapted this program with its Stimulating Access to Research in Residency (StARR) program.

Dr. Ajijola clarified that STAR was not originally conceived with a diversity focus. Twelve percent of current trainees and 10 percent of graduates self-identify as an underrepresented minority. STAR is now developing a model for postgraduate medical trainees to increase underrepresented minority representation in physician-scientist careers. In conclusion, Dr. Ajijola said, "To diversify the workforce, we should get away from thinking about pipelines to a more flexible model of highways or pathways that allow people to be recaptured."

Dr. Lewis agreed with the need to help people get back on track, rather than lose the talent through attrition. She asked for ideas about combating the financial issues that many underrepresented minorities face. Dr. Ajijola responded that investment is required to pay trainees an instructor-level rather than a graduate student salary. "Financial pressures are a huge cause for attrition and have to be addressed with investment." He noted the faculty at the UCLA Department of Medicine have committed to supporting these trainees through clinical funds and philanthropy. In response to a question from Dr. Lewis about how to convince an institution that the financial investment is worth it, Dr. Ajijola said many graduates of the program are now on the UCLA faculty. Those who have been through it are now leaders, so the case is clear. In addition, data show that recruiting talented candidates who successfully apply for external funding brings the department and university up as a whole.

DISCUSSION

Dr. Reede agreed with the need for data that go beyond numbers to the impact of participants on the institution and the discipline. It is important to learn how to better capture indirect contributions such as reputation, positioning, and leadership and to understand intra-organizational barriers and facilitators. Sharing data and spreading the word about successes is also important, she added.

A participant asked how to attract African American men at the middle school level to lead them to successful careers. Dr. Ajijola pointed to the importance of race concordance between teachers and students. Also, although money is not the cure-all, increased public school funding is needed for programs and better teacher-student ratios, he added. In addition to government action, Dr. Reede suggested taking action within professions and organizations. "We can use our influence and political power to reinforce and support the K–12 educational system and advocate for supplies, exciting curricula, and well-prepared teachers. We can link to classrooms and offer mentoring." As an example, she said the group Black Men in Medicine visits schools and talks to students.[2] Partnering with schools and community organizations and groups helps change happen on both a policy and a more granular level.

Dr. Ajijola acknowledged that the length of training time is a negative factor for some potential physician-scientists. For some underrepresented minorities, a further negative factor is not seeing professionals who look like them, he added. As positive reinforcement, many minority physician-scientists are motivated by a role model, as he was as a second-year medical student. The concept of providing young people with diverse role models is behind Mentoring in Medicine, led by Roundtable member Dr. Lynne Holden.[3]

REFERENCES

Cora-Bramble, D., K. Zhang, and L. Castillo-Page. 2010. Minority faculty members' resilience and academic productivity: Are they related? *Academic Medicine* 85: 1492–1498.

Sy, T., S. Tram-Quan, and A. Leung. 2017. Developing minority leaders: Key success factors of Asian Americans. *Asian American Journal of Psychology.* DOI: 10.1037/aap0000075.

Weber-Main, A. M., R. McGee, K. E. Boman, J. Hemming, M. Hall, T. Unold, E. M. Harwood, L. E. Risner, A. Smith, K. Lawson, J. Engler, C. J. Steer, D. Buchwald, H. P. Jones, S. O. Manson, E. Ofili, N. B. Schwartz, J. K. Vishwanatha, and K. S. Okuyemi. 2020. Grant application outcomes for biomedical researchers who participated in the National Research Mentoring Network's Grant Writing Coaching Programs. *PLOS One.* https://doi.org/10.1371/journal.pone.0241851.

Wong, M. D., L. Guerrero, T. Sallam, J. S. Frank, A. M. Fogelman, and L. L. Demer. 2016. Outcomes of a novel training program for physician-scientists: Integrating graduate degree training with specialty fellowship. *Journal of Graduate Medical Education* 8(1): 85–90. https://doi.org/10.4300/JGME-D-15-00135.1.

---

[2] See https://www.blackmeninmed.com.

[3] See http://medicalmentor.org.

7

Leadership and Organizational Solutions

In the final session of the workshop, breakout groups were each given a question tied to a short vignette and asked to discuss solutions to the issues raised. Spokespeople from the breakout groups reported back to the full workshop, followed by brief closing remarks by workshop co-chairs Dr. Randall Morgan and Dr. Joan Reede, and by Roundtable chair Dr. Cato Laurencin.

BREAKOUT GROUPS

How can a career in a dysfunctional organization be salvaged?

One group responded to a case study about an African American woman newly appointed as the CEO and president of a Boston-based nonprofit. In their vignette, after a merger between two organizations about 5 years earlier, the organization suffered from a lack of unity, an unclear mission, and financial challenges.

According to group spokesperson Delia Shelton, the group suggested looking at the root causes of the organization's problems starting with a financial perspective to show how it is losing money by not using Black talent. The CEO could reverse the organization's debt by making an argument to stakeholders so they would invest in talent and build a network of support with partners. A professional facilitator or outside panel could be brought in to increase communications within the organization. Tiffany

Reid added that the group suggested an advisory committee of people committed to the cause and to better assess existing resiliency and networks.

How should work related to advancing mentoring, diversity, and equity be recognized and rewarded?

Two groups considered this question based on a vignette about an associate professor who had formally and informally mentored many people and headed her department's Diversity, Equity, and Inclusion (DEI) committee, but whose own CV seemed bare compared with her colleagues, as explained by spokesperson Monica Hall. Marina Litvin added that the group noted the irony in which the professor supported other people but had a hard time bolstering her own case for advancement. She said the group organized their ideas into three categories: (1) organize her work with tangible results for her CV (e.g., quantify the number of mentees and their outcomes, consider publications about her mentoring results); (2) gain buy-in from her institution (show that her goals align with theirs, connect with others doing similar work across the institution to have a louder voice, mentees could amplify the results of her work); and (3) leverage external resources (applying for grants to provide support for her programs to show her work is bringing money into the institution).

Roundtable member Dr. Orlando Kirton said the second group also suggested finding metrics to attach to the mentoring activities, such as those related to the advancement of the mentees. They also observed the institution should change its value system related to promotion and that networking to pool resources and self-advocacy could change the conversation. Roundtable member Dr. Lynne Holden commented that it often requires focus and innovation to assist others but also pursue one's own goals toward advancement. She also suggested asking for mentorship help in packaging promotion materials. Walter Conwell commented on the need to "change the narrative from a 'minority tax' to 'minority capital'" from both the individual and the institutional standpoints. This might mean publishing in scholarly journals about mentoring and other work, as well as being at the table when decisions are made about which activities are valued.

How can an individual deal with transitions?

This vignette involved an accomplished surgical oncologist who accepted a leadership opportunity as an associate vice president within his institution but realizes he may have difficulties in succeeding in the position. The breakout group suggested ideas to pursue at various stages in the transition, according to Ashley Butler. Before the new position goes into effect, he could consult with people in that role or in similar positions elsewhere to better understand what the position entails and what skills are required. A barrier may be lack of confidence or self-efficacy in a new role, and an executive coach can develop necessary skills. Administrative support may help with some tasks that would allow for more focus on the big-picture demands of the position. If it does not feel like the right position after a certain period of time, he should think of an exit strategy that does not burn bridges. Workshop co-chair Dr. Reede and breakout group member Benita Wolff commented on the challenges for clinicians who find they want to stay connected to the world of practice. If that is the case, he may need to give up clinic or negotiate the time to continue some clinical work in the new position. Dr. Kirton noted even the most talented individuals have to recognize the limit to their bandwidth, or they risk failing at the edges. Dr. Morgan and Dr. Reede noted this extends not only to academic positions but also to external voluntary positions and personal life. Related to starting any new position, Dr. Reede observed that it is important to identify a mentor, coach, or sponsor to succeed. It is also important to think about the path of a new position to what comes after it and sets up for the next stage.

How can mentoring, coaching, and sponsorship for early-career professionals be advanced?

In this vignette, an assistant professor realized that mentorship and sponsorship can help in her career but does not know how to access that support. Drawing on some of the topics raised during the workshop, Marquita Hicks said the group suggested the faculty member first figure out her needs for a mentor and/or a sponsor, and recognize that preventive hesitation or defensiveness or self-doubt may impede her. She should also recognize that no one person will fill all her needs and that she may need to make herself visible so that someone wants to invest their time.

In terms of creating a supportive environment so people are more willing and positioned to mentor and sponsor, suggestions included financial incentives offered by departments as well as the requirement that a person is expected to be a mentor as part of their own advancement. Dr. Reede added that each person has individual needs; there is no one-size-fits-all type of mentorship or sponsorship. Mentors can help in identifying sponsors by vouching for their mentees. Institutions can also make mentorship and sponsorship matter by setting them up as an expectation.

Related to recruitment and advancement, workshop participant Dr. Valerae Lewis noted that at her institution, some departments are more diverse than others. They are discussing the idea of recruitment of underrepresented minorities as part of department chairs' annual assessments. Advancement is also important in addition to recruitment, added Dr. Reede. Recruitment, inclusion, and advancement are all necessary as a "triple-edged sword," commented Dr. Lewis. Several participants commented that people will move to different institutions and geographic areas if the right supports are in place.

CONCLUDING REMARKS

Dr. Morgan thanked Dr. Laura Morgan Roberts and Dr. Victoria Winston for the first vignette, which they wrote as a Harvard Business School case study, and Dr. Lewis for creating the other vignettes. He also thanked participants, the planning committee, and the staff of the National Academies for a successful workshop. Dr. Reede said she appreciated the workshop's focus on extending the arc of discussion beyond graduation to successful transitions across careers at the individual, institutional, and structural levels. Issues related to the pairing of mentors and mentees, building long-term relationships, building trust, and planning not just for tomorrow but beyond were also of importance. She thanked the representatives of new, revised, and long-standing programs for their insights about what works and what does not. Dr. Laurencin added his appreciation for a powerful and well-organized workshop.

Appendix A

Workshop Agenda

DECEMBER 7-8, 2020

Day One—December 7, 2020

9:30 AM **OPENING REMARKS**
John L. Anderson, PhD
President, National Academy of Engineering and Vice Chairman, National Research Council

Cato T. Laurencin, MD, PhD
Chair of the Roundtable; Albert and Wilda Van Dusen Distinguished Professor of Orthopaedic Surgery; Professor of Chemical and Biomolecular Engineering
Professor of Materials Science and Engineering, University of Connecticut

Randall C. Morgan, Jr., MD, MBA
Co-Chair of the Mentoring and Advising Action Group; President and CEO, Cobb/NMA Health Institute; Clinical Associate Professor of Orthopedic Surgery at Florida State School of Medicine and Clinical Associate Professor in the Department of Community Medicine, University of Connecticut

Joan Y. Reede, MD, MPH, MS, MBA
Co-Chair of the Mentoring and Advising Action Group; Professor of Medicine; Dean for Diversity and Community Partnership, Harvard Medical School: Professor in the Department of Social and Behavioral Sciences, Harvard TH Chan School of Public Health

SESSION I: UNDERSTANDING THE CURRENT STATUS OF BLACK PROFESSIONALS IN ACADEMIA AND INDUSTRY

10:00 AM **MODERATOR:**
L. D. Britt, MD, MPH, DSc(Hon), FACS, FCCM
Chairman, Surgery Department, Eastern Virginia Medical School

SPEAKERS:
Norma Poll-Hunter, PhD
Senior Director, Human Capital Initiatives; Deputy Director, Summer Medical and Dental Education Program; Diversity Policy and Programs, Association of American Medical Colleges

Karl W. Reid, EdD
Executive Director, National Society of Black Engineers; Co-Founder, the 50k Coalition; Former Associate Dean of Undergraduate Education, Massachusetts Institute of Technology

QUESTION:
What are the stats around Black STEM Professionals at various stages of transition from training to leadership?

10:30 AM **Discussion**

SESSION II: ENSURING THE ADVANCEMENT AND PROMOTION OF BLACK FACULTY

10:45 AM **MODERATOR:**

MaCalus V. Hogan, MD, MBA
Vice Chair of Education and Residency Program Director, Department of Orthopaedic Surgery; Senior Medical Director for Orthopaedic and Musculoskeletal Services, Associate Professor, University of Pittsburgh Medical Center

SPEAKERS:

George Q. Daley, MD, PhD
Dean of Faculty and Caroline Shields Walker Professor of Medicine, Harvard Medical School

Augustine M. K. Choi, MD
Stephen and Suzanne Weiss Dean, Weill Cornell Medicine and Provost for Medical Affairs, Cornell University

Deborah Prothrow-Stith, MD1
Dean and Professor of Medicine, College of Medicine, Charles R. Drew University of Medicine and Science

Gilda A. Barabino, PhD
President and Professor of Biomedical and Chemical Engineering, Olin College of Engineering

QUESTION:
How are Presidents and Deans helping to advance Black faculty leadership and promotion in their institutions?

11:45 AM **Discussion**

12:15 PM **Break for Lunch**

[1] Did not attend or present.

SESSION III: MENTOR-MENTEE CONVERSATIONS

12:45 PM **MODERATOR:**

Wendy L. Yallowitz, MSW
Senior Program Officer, Robert Wood Johnson Foundation

Mentor: Kafui Dzirasa, MD, PhD
Associate Professor of Psychiatry and Behavioral Sciences; K. Ranga Rama Krishnan Associate Professor, Duke University School of Medicine

Mentee: Aza Allsop, MD, PhD
Psychiatry Resident, NRTP, Department of Psychiatry, Yale University School of Medicine

Mentor: Eve J. Higginbotham, SM, MD
Vice Dean for Inclusion and Diversity, Perelman School of Medicine; Professor, Ophthalmology, Perelman School of Medicine

Mentee: Ahmara G. Ross, MD, PhD
Assistant Professor, Ophthalmology, Hospital of the University of Pennsylvania; Assistant Professor of Neurology

Mentor: Gilda A. Barabino, PhD
Professor of Biomedical and Chemical Engineering and President, Olin College of Engineering

Mentee: Shereka Banton, PhD
Senior Regulatory Affairs Program Lead, Johnson & Johnson

QUESTIONS:

- What are challenges to mentor-mentee interactions?
- What are best practices/lessons learned from your experience?
- How did the mentoring relationship begin and what are changes through career transitions?

1:45 PM **Discussion**

2:15 PM **Break**

SESSION IV: SOCIAL SCIENCE – WHAT IS NEEDED?

2:30 PM **MODERATOR:**

Orlando C. Kirton, MD, MBA
Surgeon-in-Chief, Chairman of Surgery, Abington-Jefferson Health
Chief Division of General Surgery, Abington-Jefferson Health
Vice Chairman, Jefferson Health Enterprise Department of Surgery
Professor of Surgery, Sidney Kimmel Medical College of Thomas Jefferson University

SPEAKERS:

Stacy Blake-Beard, PhD
Visiting Professor, Tuck School of Business at Dartmouth; Faculty Program Chair, Simmons College Executive Education
Mentoring, Coaching and Sponsorship: Sources of Critical Support and Feedback

Laura Morgan Roberts, PhD
Professor of Practice, University of Virginia Darden School of Business
Toward a racially just workplace: Advancing true inclusion for people with diverse talents

QUESTIONS:

- Describe the relationships and the intersection of roles in mentorship, coaching, and sponsorship?
- Describe organizational change to attract and retain diverse talent?

3:30 PM **Discussion**

4:00 PM **Wrap-up**

4:30 PM **Day One Adjourned**

Day Two—December 8, 2020

SESSION V: PROGRAM MODELS AND BEST PRACTICES

1:15 PM **MODERATOR:**
Valerae O. Lewis, MD
Professor and Chair, Department of Orthopaedic Oncology; Director, Orthopaedic Center; Associate Director of the Sarcoma Center, University of Texas MD Anderson Cancer Center

SPEAKERS:
Nina Ardery
Deputy Director, Harold Amos Medical Faculty Development Program (AMFDP), Robert Wood Johnson Foundation

Elizabeth O. Ofili, MD, MPH, FACC
Professor of Medicine; Director and Senior Associate Dean, Clinical Research Center and Clinical Translational Research, Morehouse School of Medicine

Joan Y. Reede, MD, MPH, MS, MBA
Co-Chair of the Mentoring and Advising Action Group; Professor of Medicine; Dean for Diversity and Community Partnership, Harvard Medical School: Professor in the Department of Social and Behavioral Sciences, Harvard TH Chan School of Public Health

Olujimi Ajijola, MD, PhD
Assistant Professor of Medicine, UCLA Cardiac Arrhythmia Center, David Geffen School of Medicine; Director of the Clinical Autonomic Neuroscience Programs, and Autonomic Testing Laboratory, University of California Los Angeles

QUESTIONS:
- What are your best practices and outcomes?
- What lessons can be learned for scaling?

2:15 PM **Discussion**

SESSION VI: LEADERSHIP AND ORGANIZATIONAL SOLUTIONS (BREAKOUT ROOMS)

2:30 PM **QUESTION 1:**
- How to Salvage a Career in a Dysfunctional Organization?

MODERATOR:
Randall C. Morgan, Jr., MD, MBA
Co-Chair of the Mentoring and Advising Action Group; President and CEO, Cobb/NMA Health Institute; Clinical Associate Professor of Orthopedic Surgery at Florida State School of Medicine and Clinical Associate Professor in the Department of Community Medicine at the University of Connecticut

QUESTION 2:
- How to Recognize and Reward Work Related to Advancing Mentoring, Diversity, and Equity?

MODERATORS:
Monica Hall
Program Associate, Robert Wood Johnson Foundation

Orlando C. Kirton, MD, MBA
Surgeon-in-Chief, Chairman of Surgery, Abington-Jefferson Health
Chief Division of General Surgery, Abington-Jefferson Health
Vice Chairman, Jefferson Health Enterprise Department of Surgery
Professor of Surgery, Sidney Kimmel Medical College of Thomas Jefferson University

QUESTION 3:
- How to Deal with Transitions?

MODERATOR:
Lynne M. Holden, MD
Professor, Department of Emergency Medicine, Albert Einstein College of Medicine

QUESTION 4:
- How to Advance Mentoring, Coaching and Sponsorship for Early-Career Professionals?

MODERATORS:
Joan Y. Reede, MD, MPH, MS, MBA
Co-Chair of the Mentoring and Advising Action Group; Professor of Medicine; Dean for Diversity and Community Partnership, Harvard Medical School: Professor in the Department of Social and Behavioral Sciences, Harvard TH Chan School of Public Health l

Valerae O. Lewis, MD
Professor and Chair, Department of Orthopaedic Oncology; Director, Orthopaedic Center; Associate Director of the Sarcoma Center, University of Texas MD Anderson Cancer Center

3:00 PM	**Report from Breakout Rooms** Moderator: Randall C. Morgan, Jr., MD, MBA
4:00 PM	**Closing Discussion and Remarks**
4:30 PM	**Day Two Adjourned**

Appendix B

Biographical Sketches of Presenters

John L. Anderson, Ph.D., has been president of the National Academy of Engineering (NAE) since July 1, 2019. He was born in Wilmington, Delaware, and received his undergraduate degree from the University of Delaware in 1967 and Ph.D. degree from the University of Illinois at Urbana-Champaign in 1971, both in chemical engineering. He was most recently Distinguished Professor of Chemical Engineering and president (2007–2015) of the Illinois Institute of Technology (IIT). Before that he was provost and executive vice president at Case Western Reserve University (2004–2007), following 28 years at Carnegie Mellon University, including 8 years as dean of the College of Engineering and 11 years as head of the Chemical Engineering Department. He began his professional career as an assistant professor of chemical engineering at Cornell University (1971–1976).

Dr. Anderson was elected to the NAE in 1992 for contributions to the understanding of colloidal hydrodynamics and membrane transport phenomena and was elected an NAE councillor in 2015. His service also includes numerous National Academies activities, such as the Committee on Determining Basic Research Needs to Interrupt the Improvised Explosive Device Delivery Chain (chair); Committee on Review of Existing and Potential Standoff Explosives Detection Techniques (chair); Organizing Committee for the National Security and Homeland Defense Workshop (co-chair); Board on Chemical Sciences and Technology (co-chair); and

Ford Foundation Minority Postdoctoral Review Panel on Physical Sciences, Mathematics, and Engineering.

In addition to his NAE membership, Dr. Anderson is a fellow of the American Academy of Arts and Sciences and the American Association for the Advancement of Science. He was appointed to the National Science Board in 2014 for a 6-year term. He received the Acrivos Professional Progress Award from the American Institute of Chemical Engineers (AIChE) and an award from the Pittsburgh Section of AIChE for "Outstanding Professional Accomplishments in the Field of Academics," and he is listed on the Alumni Wall of Fame at the University of Delaware. In 2012, he received the National Engineering Award from the American Association of Engineering Societies. He has held visiting professorships at the Massachusetts Institute of Technology (fellow of the John Simon Guggenheim Foundation), University of Melbourne (Australia), and Landbouwuniversiteit Wageningen (the Netherlands). He has presented guest lectures at universities throughout the United States and is the author of numerous journal articles and book chapters.

Cato T. Laurencin, M.D., Ph.D. (NAM, NAE) *(Chair)*, is the University Professor and Albert and Wilda Van Dusen Distinguished Endowed Professor of Orthopaedic Surgery at the University of Connecticut (UConn). He is professor of chemical engineering, professor of materials science and engineering, and professor of biomedical engineering at the school. He serves as the chief executive officer of the Connecticut Convergence Institute for Translation in Regenerative Engineering and the director of the Raymond and Beverly Sackler Center for Biomedical, Biological, Physical and Engineering Sciences at UConn.

Dr. Laurencin earned a B.S.E. in chemical engineering from Princeton University, and his M.D., magna cum laude, from Harvard Medical School, and received the Robinson Award for Surgery. He earned his Ph.D. in biochemical engineering/biotechnology from the Massachusetts Institute of Technology, where he was named a Hugh Hampton Young fellow. A practicing sports medicine and shoulder surgeon, Dr. Laurencin has been named to America's Top Doctors for more than 15 years. He is a fellow of the American Academy of Orthopaedic Surgeons, a fellow of the American Orthopaedic Association, a fellow of the American College of Surgeons, and a member of the American Surgical Association. He received the Nicolas Andry Award, the highest honor of the Association of Bone and Joint Surgeons. Dr. Laurencin served as dean of the Medical School and vice president for health affairs at the University of Connecticut.

Dr. Laurencin is a pioneer of the new field of Regenerative Engineering. He is an expert in biomaterials science, stem cell technology, and nanotechnology and was named one of the 100 Engineers of the Modern Era by the American Institute of Chemical Engineers. He received the Founder's Award (highest award) from the Society for Biomaterials, the Von Hipple Award (highest award) from the Materials Research Society, and the James Bailey Award (highest award) from the Society for Biological Engineering. He received the National Institutes of Health (NIH) Director's Pioneer Award, NIH's highest and most prestigious research award, for his new field of Regenerative Engineering and the National Science Foundation's Emerging Frontiers in Research and Innovation Grant Award. Dr. Laurencin is the editor-in-chief of *Regenerative Engineering and Translational Medicine*, published by Springer Nature, and is the founder of the Regenerative Engineering Society. He is a fellow of the American Chemical Society, the American Institute of Chemical Engineers, the Biomedical Engineering Society, the Materials Research Society, and the American Association for the Advancement of Science (AAAS). The AAAS awarded Dr. Laurencin the Philip Hauge Abelson Prize given "for signal contributions to the advancement of science in the United States."

Dr. Laurencin is active in mentoring, especially underrepresented minority students. He received the AAAS Mentor Award, the Beckman Award for Mentoring, and the Presidential Award for Excellence in Science, Math and Engineering Mentoring in ceremonies at the White House. The Society for Biomaterials established the Cato T. Laurencin, M.D., Ph.D. Travel Fellowship in his honor, awarded to underrepresented minority students pursuing research. Dr. Laurencin is also active in addressing health disparities. Dr. Laurencin completed the Program in African American Studies at Princeton University. He is a core faculty member of the Africana Studies Institute at the University of Connecticut, and is editor-in-chief of the *Journal of Racial and Ethnic Health Disparities*, published by Springer Nature. He co-founded the W. Montague Cobb/NMA Health Institute, dedicated to addressing health disparities, and served as its founding chair. The W. Montague Cobb/NMA Health Institute and the National Medical Association established the Cato T. Laurencin Lifetime Research Achievement Award, given during the opening ceremonies of the National Medical Association Meeting. He is a recipient of the Herbert W. Nickens Award from AAAS recognizing his work advancing social justice and equity.

Dr. Laurencin is an elected member of the National Academy of Medicine, an elected member of the National Academy of Engineering, and an elected member of the American Academy of Arts and Sciences. Active internationally, he is an elected fellow of the Indian National Academy of Sciences, the Indian National Academy of Engineering, the African Academy of Sciences, and the World Academy of Sciences, and is an academician of the Chinese Academy of Engineering.

Dr. Laurencin is the recipient of the National Medal of Technology and Innovation, America's highest honor for technological achievement, awarded by President Barack Obama in ceremonies at the White House. He is the first individual in history to receive the oldest/highest award of the National Academy of Medicine (the Walsh McDermott Medal) and the oldest, highest award of the National Academy of Engineering (the Simon Ramo Founder's Award).

Randall C. Morgan, Jr., M.D., M.B.A., is the president and CEO of the W. Montague Cobb/NMA Health Institute based in Washington, D.C. In that role he leads a staff of scholars and research specialists who focus upon the elimination of health disparities. He is also an active orthopedic surgeon who has practiced in Sarasota and Bradenton, Florida, since 2005. He serves as founder and president of University Park Orthopedics in that community. He is clinical associate professor of orthopedic surgery at Florida State School of Medicine and clinical associate professor in the Department of Community Medicine at the University of Connecticut. He is a graduate of Grinnell College with a B.A. in chemistry. He received his M.D. degree from Howard University. He served as a resident in orthopedic surgery at Northwestern University and served a Pediatric Orthopedic Fellowship at Children's Hospital in Cincinnati. He later received an M.B.A. degree from the University of South Florida.

Dr. Morgan served as the 95th president of the National Medical Association during 1996 and 1997. He was the first board-certified orthopedic surgeon to hold that position. Dr. Morgan is a true pioneer in his profession and was among the first surgeons to perform total joint replacement surgery at Northwestern University. Dr. Morgan has practiced general orthopedic surgery and pediatric orthopedics in Evanston, Illinois, as well in his hometown of Gary, Indiana, for more than 30 years prior to his relocation to Sarasota. With the assistance of his father, Mr. Randall C. Morgan, Sr., he founded the Orthopedic Centers of Northwest Indiana and served as its president from 1975 to 1999. At one time, this was the largest minority-owned orthopedic practice in the United States. He has written and published extensively throughout his career on orthopedics, social responsibility, health equity and the education pipeline for underrepresented young scholars. He is a diplomat of the American Board of Orthopedic Surgery and the American Board of Managed Care Medicine. He is also a fellow of the American College of Surgeons and a member of Alpha Omega Alpha honorary medical society.

Joan Y. Reede, M.D., M.P.H., M.S., M.B.A., is the dean for diversity and community partnership and professor of medicine at Harvard Medical School (HMS). Dr. Reede also holds appointments as professor in the Department of Social and Behavioral Sciences at the Harvard T. H. Chan School of Public Health, and is an assistant in health policy at Massachusetts General Hospital. Dr. Reede is responsible for the development and management of a comprehensive program that provides leadership, guidance, and support to promote the increased recruitment, retention, and advancement of underrepresented minority, women, LGBT, and faculty with disabilities at HMS. This charge includes oversight of all diversity activities at HMS as they relate to faculty, trainees, students, and staff. Dr. Reede also serves as the director of the Minority Faculty Development Program, program director of the Faculty Diversity Program of the Harvard Catalyst/Harvard Clinical and Translational Science Center, and chair of the HMS Task Force on Diversity and Inclusion. Dr. Reede has served on a number of boards and committees including the Secretary's Advisory Committee to the Director of the National Institutes of Health (NIH); the Sullivan Commission on Diversity in the Healthcare Workforce; the National Children's Study Advisory Committee of the *Eunice Kennedy Shriver* National Institute of Child Health and Human Development; and the Advisory Committee to the Deputy Director for Intramural Research of NIH. Some of her past affiliations include the Steering Committee and Task Force for the Annual Biomedical Research Conference for Minority Students (ABRCMS); past co-chair of the Bias Review Committee of the Advisory Committee to the NIH Director's Working Group on Diversity; the Association of American Medical Colleges (AAMC) Careers in Medicine Committee; and past chair of the AAMC Group on Diversity and Inclusion (GDI). Dr. Reede served on the editorial board of the *American Journal of Public Health*, and she was the guest editor for the AAMC 2012 special issue *Diversity and Inclusion in Academic Medicine* of *Academic Medicine*. She is a past chair of the National Academy of Medicine's Interest Group 08 on Health of Populations/Health

Disparities. In 2018, Dr. Reede was appointed to the National Advisory Council on Minority Health and Health Disparities (NACMHD). Dr. Reede is an authority in the area of workforce development and diversity. Her colleagues and mentees have recognized her with a number of awards that include the Herbert W. Nickens Award from AAMC and the Society of General Medicine in 2005; election to the National Academy of Medicine in 2009; the 2011 Diversity Award from the Association of University Professors; and in 2012 she was the recipient of an Elizabeth Hurlock Beckman Trust Award. In 2013 she received an Exemplar STEM Award from the Urban Education Institute at North Carolina A&T University in Greensboro, North Carolina, and in 2015, she was the Distinguished Woman Scientist and Scholar ADVANCE Lecturer at the University of Maryland School of Public Health. Dr. Reede was recognized by her medical school classmates as a recipient of the Mount Sinai Alumni Association and Icahn School of Medicine 2015 Jacobi Medallion for extraordinary leaders in health care, and in 2017 she was nominated by her peers and received a Harvard T. H. Chan School of Public Health Alumni Award.

L. D. Britt, M.D., M.P.H., D.Sc. (Hon.), F.A.C.S., F.C.C.M., a proud native of Suffolk, Virginia, and a member of the National Academy of Medicine, has strong southern roots and is the product of the public school system. Dr. Britt, a graduate of Harvard Medical School and Harvard School of Public Health, is the Brickhouse Professor and Chairman of the Department of Surgery at Eastern Virginia Medical School. He is the author of 300 scientific publications (with more than 231 being peer-reviewed articles). In addition, he is the author of three textbooks, including a recent edition of the highly touted *Acute Care Surgery* (Lippincott, Williams & Wilkens, Medford, NJ). He serves on numerous editorial boards, including the *Annals of Surgery*; *Archives of Surgery*; *World Journal of Surgery*; *Journal of the American College of Surgeons*; *American Journal of Surgery* (associate editor); *Journal of Emergency, Trauma, and Shock*; *Journal of Surgical Education*; *American Surgeon*; and others. In addition, he is a reviewer for the *New England Journal of Medicine*. Dr. Britt, a member of Alpha Omega Alpha, is the recipient of the nation's highest teaching award in medicine—the Robert J. Glaser Distinguished Teaching Award, which is given by the Association of American Medical Colleges in conjunction with the American Orthopaedic Association. He was honored by the Association of Surgical Education with its lifetime achievement award—the Distinguished Educator Award—given annually to one person considered by his peers to be a true master. More than 200 institutions throughout the world have invited him to be their distinguished visiting professor. He was recently the William P. Longmire, M.D., Visiting Professor at the University of California, Los Angeles. Dr. Britt is the past president of the Society of Surgical Chairs and the past chairman of the Accreditation Council for Graduate Medical Education Residency Review Committee for Surgery. In addition, he is the past secretary of the Southern Surgical Association, the past recorder/program chair for the American Association for the Surgery of Trauma, and past president of the Southeastern Surgical Congress, the Halsted Society, and the Southern Surgical Association. Dr. Britt is the past chairman of the Board of Regents of the American College of Surgeons. He is also the past president of the American College of Surgeons, the American Association for the Surgery of Trauma, and the American Surgical Association. At the inaugural presidential ceremony held in Washington, D.C., during the 96th annual Clinical Congress of the American College of Surgeons, Dr. Britt was awarded the U.S. Surgeon General's medallion for his outstanding achievements in medicine. The National Library of Medicine of the National Institutes of Health (in collaboration with the Reginald F. Lewis Museum of Maryland African American History and Culture) featured Dr. Britt for his contributions to academic surgery. President George W. Bush recognized Dr. Britt's leadership role in medicine and nominated him to the Board of Regents of the Uniformed Services University (confirmed by the United States Senate). At the end of his tenure, Dr. Britt was awarded the Distinguished Service Medal.

An active participant in the community, Dr. Britt has received numerous awards for public service. Dr. Britt is the recipient of the 2010 Colgate Darden Citizen of the Year Award and the 2011 Dr. Martin Luther King, Jr. Community Award. The *Atlanta Post* recently highlighted him as one of the top 21 Black doctors in America. At the 2012 annual meeting of the American Surgical Association, Dr. Britt became the 132nd president of the organization. He was conferred an honorary doctorate by the president of Tuskegee University. Dr. Britt was also elected to the position of commissioner of the Joint Commission (formerly JACHO). In 2012, he was conferred an Honorary Fellowship in the French Academy of Surgery, and the Colleges of Medicine of South Africa. Having recently been awarded an Honorary Fellowship in the Royal College of Surgeons of Glasgow, Dr. Britt now has the distinction of receiving the highest honor given by each of the four Royal Colleges in the United Kingdom—England, Edinburg, Ireland, and Glasgow.

In addition to the unveiling of his latest edition of the textbook *Acute Care Surgery* (Wolters Kluwer), Dr. Britt was inducted into the inaugural class of the Academy of Master Surgeons Educators of the American College of Surgeons in October 2018. He is a founding member of the Academy. In 2019, Dr. Britt was awarded the coveted Silbergleit Award given by the Association of Program Directors in Surgery. He is only the third individual to receive this recognition for his sustained leadership role as an accomplished program director.

Norma Poll-Hunter, Ph.D., is the senior director of Human Capital Initiatives within Diversity Policy and Programs at the Association of American Medical Colleges (AAMC). In this role, she leads a portfolio of career development programs with a focus on diversity and inclusion across the medical education continuum. She serves as the deputy director for the Summer Health Professions Education Program, a national pipeline program to increase diversity in the health professions. She also leads initiatives focused on cultural competence in medical education, building collaborations and partnerships to advance diversity, and research and evaluation projects focused on diversity in the health-care workforce. Prior to the AAMC, Dr. Poll-Hunter practiced as a bilingual psychologist at a regional hospital in Upstate New York. Following receipt of her B.A. from Lehman College, City University of New York, Dr. Poll-Hunter earned her Ph.D. in counseling psychology at the University of Albany, State University of New York.

Karl W. Reid, Ed.D., was named executive director of the National Society of Black Engineers (NSBE) on June 2, 2014, marking his return to the organization that gave him his first major leadership experience, 32 years earlier. For the past 22 years, he has been a leading advocate for increasing college access, opportunity, and success for low-income and minority youth. Dr. Reid went to NSBE from the United Negro College Fund (UNCF), where he oversaw new program development, research, and capacity building for the organization's 37 historically black colleges and universities and held the title of senior vice president for research, innovation, and member college engagement. Before his service at UNCF, he worked in positions of progressive responsibility to increase diversity at his alma mater, the Massachusetts Institute of Technology (MIT), which he left as associate dean of undergraduate education and director of the Office of Minority Education. While working at MIT as director of Engineering Outreach Programs, Dr. Reid earned his doctor of education degree at Harvard University. His dissertation explored the interrelationship of race, identity, and academic achievement. He is the author of *Working Smarter, Not Just Harder: Three Sensible Strategies for Succeeding in College ... and Life*.

Dr. Reid was born in the Bronx, New York, and grew up in Roosevelt, New York, a mostly working-class, African American community on Long Island. The high value his parents placed on education, and his admission to a well-resourced, magnet high school near Roosevelt, put him on a track to follow his older brother to MIT, where he earned his undergraduate and master's degrees in materials science and engineering and was a Tau Beta Pi Scholar. He credits his membership in the NSBE chapter at MIT with giving a vital boost to his self-confidence and leadership skills. He joined the society during his freshman year, was elected chapter vice president his junior year, and subsequently served as NSBE national chairperson.

After graduating from MIT, Dr. Reid worked in the computer industry for 12 years, in product management, marketing, sales, and consulting. In 1991, 5 years into a successful career in sales and marketing with the IBM Corporation, Dr. Reid read Jonathan Kozol's *Savage Inequalities*, a seminal book about educational disparities in the United States, which sparked his passion for bringing about positive change through education of African Americans and other underserved populations.

Dr. Reid sits on the DC STEM Council, the Dean's Advisory Cabinet of the Harvard University School of Engineering and Applied Sciences, as well as the Dean's Advisory Council for Diversity, Equity and Inclusion at the University of Michigan College of Engineering. He holds memberships in the American Association of Engineering Societies, the American Society of Engineering Education, and the Council of Engineering and Scientific Society Executives. Dr. Reid is also a founding member of the 50k Coalition, a national effort to produce 50,000 diverse engineering graduates annually by 2025. He was recently named a Top 100 Executive in America by *Uptown Professional* magazine. He is a frequent contributor to the national diversity engineering dialogue, author of several commentary pieces, and quoted in numerous articles in publications such as *Forbes*, *The Wall Street Journal*, *U.S. News & World Report*, and *The Hechinger Report*.

Dr. Reid is now supporting NSBE's National Executive Board and the Society's 25,000 active members in reaching the main goal of NSBE's 10-year Strategic Plan: to end the underrepresentation of Blacks in engineering in the United States by annually producing 10,000 Black engineers in the country, by 2025.

MaCalus V. Hogan, M.D., M.B.A., is the vice chair of education and Residency Program director in the Department of Orthopaedic Surgery at the University of Pittsburgh Medical Center (UPMC). He oversees all educational and training programs within the department. He is an associate professor in the Departments of Orthopaedic Surgery and Bioengineering. He completed medical school at Howard University College of Medicine in Washington, D.C. He was the recipient of a National Institutes of Health Training Grant and served as a Musculoskeletal Tissue Repair and Regeneration Research fellow at the University of Virginia Health System, Department of Orthopaedic Surgery, in Charlottesville, Virginia, where he also completed his orthopaedic surgical residency training. This was followed by a foot and ankle fellowship at the Hospital for Special Surgery in New York City. Following the completion of his training in 2013, Dr. Hogan joined UPMC.

Dr. Hogan has experience in the realm of health-care policy and quality of care delivery, currently serving as the medical director for Outcomes and Registries for the UPMC Donald F. Wolff, Jr. Center for Quality, Safety, and Innovation. He is co-chair of the UPMC Orthopaedic Bundling Advisory Board, sits on the UPMC Orthopaedic Service Line Steering Committee, and serves on the Executive Committee for the Department of Orthopaedics.

With a passion for research, Dr. Hogan's interest is in musculoskeletal regenerative medicine with a focus on tendon, ligament, and cartilage bioengineering. He is currently directing the Foot and Ankle Injury Research (F.A.I.R.) group and co-directs the Musculoskeletal Growth and Regeneration Lab. He has published more than 100 manuscripts, book chapters, and presentations. He presents both nationally and internationally on his management of foot and ankle injuries, regenerative medicine, and clinical outcomes research. In 2013, Dr. Hogan and his research team received the American Orthopaedic Foot and Ankle Society J. Leonard Goldner Award for best basic science research for their work on tendon regeneration titled "Successful Achilles Tendon Regeneration using a Bioresorbable Nanofiber Scaffold, Stem Cells, and Growth Factor in a Rat Tendon Gap Defect Model." In 2014, Dr. Hogan received the American Orthopaedic Association (AOA) Emerging Leader on the Move Award. He is a member of various professional organizations and societies, including, but not limited to, the AOA Emerging Leaders Program, the American Orthopaedic Foot and Ankle Society, the Orthopaedic Research Society, and the American Academy of Orthopaedic Surgeons. He and his research team were named

New Investigator Recognition Award Finalists by the Orthopaedic Research Society in both 2013 and 2015. Dr. Hogan serves as a foot and ankle consultant for the athletic departments at the University of Pittsburgh, Carnegie Mellon University, and Duquesne University, and also serves as the Assistant Team Physician for Point Park University and the Conservatory of Performing Arts.

In the fall of 2017, Dr. Hogan served as an AOA North American Traveling fellow, a highly competitive program that promotes clinical and scientific exchange across U.S. and Canadian health systems to discuss diverse ways that leaders address challenges facing orthopaedic surgery today. Dr. Hogan has been selected by his peers as a Best Doctor in America in 2016, 2017, and 2018.

George Q. Daley, M.D., Ph.D., is dean and Caroline Shields Walker Professor of Medicine at Harvard Medical School. He is also professor of biological chemistry and molecular pharmacology. Prior to becoming dean, he was the director of the Pediatric Stem Cell Transplantation Program at Dana-Farber/Boston Children's Cancer and Blood Disorders Center and an investigator of the Howard Hughes Medical Institute. Dr. Daley received his A.B., magna cum laude, from Harvard (1982); a Ph.D. in biology from the Massachusetts Institute of Technology (1989), working with Nobel laureate David Baltimore; and his M.D., summa cum laude, from Harvard Medical School (1991). Dr. Daley pursued clinical training in internal medicine at Massachusetts General Hospital, where he served as chief resident (1994–1995), and a clinical fellowship in hematology/oncology at Brigham and Women's Hospital and Children's Hospitals. He remains a staff member in Pediatric Hematology/Oncology at Boston Children's Hospital. His research uses mouse and human disease models to study cancer and blood disorders. Dr. Daley has been elected to the National Academy of Medicine, the American Society for Clinical Investigation, the American Association of Physicians, the American Pediatric Societies, the American Academy of Arts and Sciences, and the American Association for the Advancement of Science. He was an inaugural winner of the National Institutes of Health Director's Pioneer Award (2004), and has won the E. Donnall Thomas Prize of the American Society of Hematology. He was a founding executive committee member of the Harvard Stem Cell Institute, served as president of the International Society for Stem Cell Research (2007–2008), and anchored the special task forces that produced the society's guidelines for stem cell research and clinical translation (2006,

2008, 2016). He was on the organizing committee for both the 2015 and 2018 International Summits on Human Genome Editing and has advocated publicly for responsible international guidelines for attempts at germline genome editing.

Augustine M. K. Choi, M.D., an internationally renowned physician-scientist in the field of lung disease, has focused his research on understanding how chronic and acute lung diseases develop in response to molecular, cellular, and genetic triggers. His laboratory studies how oxidative stress and inflammation affect stress response genes and antioxidant enzymes in the lung, and it has contributed much to our understanding of the molecular regulation and function of heme oxygenase-1 and gaseous molecule carbon monoxide in lung and vascular disease. Dr. Choi is currently examining whether inhaled carbon monoxide can be an effective therapy in human disease.

Dr. Choi has a longstanding commitment to the training of postdoctoral fellows and physician-scientists in lung diseases. He has published more than 350 peer-reviewed articles and is a member of the National Academy of Medicine, American Society of Clinical Investigation, and the Association of American Physicians. He is currently funded by multiple National Institutes of Health R01 grants. Among his many awards and honors are the 2011 Ho-Am Prize in Medicine, which is often referred to as the Korean Nobel Prize, and the 2015 J. Burns Amberson Lecture, which recognizes a career of major lifetime contributions to pulmonary research.

Dr. Choi received a bachelor's degree in 1980 from the University of Kentucky and an M.D. in 1984 from the University of Louisville. After completing his internship and residency in internal medicine at Duke University and a fellowship in pulmonary and critical care medicine at Johns Hopkins University, he began his academic career in 1990 in the division of pulmonary and critical care medicine at Johns Hopkins. In 1998, he moved to an appointment at Yale University, and in 2000, he became chief of the Division of Pulmonary, Allergy and Critical Care Medicine at the University of Pittsburgh. In 2007, he was appointed the Parker B. Francis Professor of Medicine at Harvard Medical School and chief of pulmonary and critical care medicine at Brigham and Women's Hospital. He served as the Sanford I. Weill Chairman and Professor of Medicine in the Joan and Sanford I. Weill Department of Medicine at Weill Cornell Medicine and as physician-in-chief of New York-Presbyterian/Weill Cornell Medical Center, prior to his appointment as dean in January 2017.

Deborah Prothrow-Stith, M.D.,[1] is dean and professor of medicine for the College of Medicine at Charles R. Drew University of Medicine and Science. Dr. Prothrow-Stith is an internationally recognized public health leader, who since 2008 has advised top-tier health-care, life sciences, academic, and not-for-profit institutions on leadership and executive talent in her role as a principal at the global executive search consulting firm Spencer Stuart. Prior to joining Spencer Stuart, she served as the Henry Pickering Walcott Professor of Public Health Practice and associate dean for diversity at the Harvard School of Public Health, where she created and led the Division of Public Health Practice, and secured more than $14 million in grant funding for public health programs.

As a physician working in inner-city Boston, Dr. Prothrow-Stith broke new ground with her efforts to define youth violence as a public health problem. She developed and wrote "The Violence Prevention Curriculum for Adolescents," a forerunner of violence prevention curricula for schools and communities. She is the author of *Deadly Consequences*, the first book to present the public health perspective on violence to a mass audience. She has authored and co-authored more than 100 publications. She is co-author of a blueprint for community-based violence prevention in *Murder Is No Accident* (Jossey Bass Publishers, 2004) and a guide for parents of adolescent girls in *Sugar and Spice and No Longer Nice* (Jossey Bass Publishers, 2005). She is also co-author of a high school health education textbook, *Health* (Pearson 2014), that is in its third publication.

In 1987, Governor Michael Dukakis appointed her the first woman commissioner of public health for Massachusetts, where she led a department with 3,500 employees, 8 hospitals, and a budget of $350 million. She established the nation's first Office of Violence Prevention in a state department of public health, expanded prevention programs for HIV/AIDS, and increased drug treatment and rehabilitation programs. Dr. Prothrow-Stith and her family lived in Tanzania during her husband's tenure as U.S. ambassador, where she worked with several local organizations, including Muhimbili National Hospital and a nongovernmental organization that runs the first HIV clinic in Tanzania.

She is a graduate of Spelman College and Harvard Medical School. She completed residency training in internal medicine at Boston City Hospital and is certified by the American Board of Internal Medicine. In 2003, Dr. Prothrow-Stith was elected to membership in the prestigious National

[1] Did not attend or present.

Academy of Medicine. She has received 10 honorary doctorates, including ones from Morehouse Medical School and Meharry Medical College. She is the recipient of the 1993 World Health Day Award, the 1989 Secretary of Health and Human Service Award, and a presidential appointment to the National Commission on Crime Control and Prevention. In 2015, she was inducted into the honor roll of women physicians in the Massachusetts Medical Society.

Gilda A. Barabino, Ph.D., became the second president of Olin College of Engineering, and professor of biomedical and chemical engineering, on July 1, 2020. Previously she served as dean of the Grove School of Engineering at the City College of New York (CCNY). She also served as Daniel and Frances Berg Professor, with appointments in the Departments of Biomedical Engineering and Chemical Engineering, as well as the City University of New York School of Medicine.

A biomedical engineer trained in chemical engineering, with broad interest in global health, systems, and interdisciplinary engineering education, Dr. Barabino is a noted investigator in the areas of sickle cell disease and cellular and tissue engineering. She is an internationally recognized thought leader and highly sought speaker and consultant on race/ethnicity and gender in science and engineering, with particular focus on creating cultures and climates that support a sense of belonging. She has led a number of initiatives in these areas, including serving as the founder and executive director of the National Institute for Faculty Equity.

Before joining CCNY, she served as associate chair for graduate studies and professor in the Wallace H. Coulter Department of Biomedical Engineering at Georgia Tech and Emory University. She also served as Georgia Tech's inaugural vice provost for academic diversity. Prior to that, she spent 18 years at Northeastern University, rising to the rank of full professor of chemical engineering and serving as vice provost for undergraduate education.

Dr. Barabino is an active member of the National Academy of Engineering and the National Academy of Medicine and serves on numerous committees of the National Academies of Sciences, Engineering, and Medicine, including the Committee on Women in Science, Engineering, and Medicine; the Roundtable on Black Men and Black Women in Science, Engineering, and Medicine; the Underrepresentation of Women of Color in Tech project; the Ad-Hoc Committee for the Gulf Scholars Program; the Committee on Addressing Sickle Cell Disease; and the National Institutes of Health National Institute of Biomedical Imaging and Bioengineering Strategic Planning Working Group. Dr. Barabino also serves as a member of the National Science Foundation's Advisory Committee for Engineering; the congressionally mandated Committee on Equal Opportunities in Science and Engineering; and the American Association for the Advancement of Science Committee on Science, Engineering and Public Policy. Dr. Barabino also serves on the Scientific Advisory Board of the Chan Zuckerberg Biohub.

Her many honors include the American Institute of Chemical Engineers Award for Service to Society (2019); the Presidential Award for Excellence in Science, Mathematics, and Engineering Mentoring (2018); the Pierre Galletti Award (2017), the American Institute for Medical and Biological Engineering's highest honor; and an honorary degree from Xavier University of Louisiana (2016). She is currently the chair of the American Society of Engineering Education Engineering Deans Council. She sits on the board of trustees for VentureWell, Associated Universities, Inc., and Xavier University of Louisiana.

Dr. Barabino earned her B.S. degree in chemistry from Xavier University of Louisiana and her Ph.D. in chemical engineering from Rice University.

Wendy L. Yallowitz, M.S.W., senior program officer, joined the Robert Wood Johnson Foundation (RWJF) in 2001, bringing her expertise in long-term care and services for older adults to the foundation's work with vulnerable populations. Drawn to RWJF by "its direction, resources, and the opportunity to make a difference," she focuses on developing programs that have an impact on individuals' health at the community level.

Ms. Yallowitz has extensive experience and knowledge in mental health, with a concentration on blending social and emotional learning into K–12 education. She specializes in long-term care strategies, such as aging in place, and home and community-based services. Her past work also included emphasis on programs that helped immigrant and refugee communities adjust to life in the United States with the supports they need to improve and maintain health. Her work expertise includes scaling successful models and identifying the feasibility of adapting these models to other populations, creating innovative programs that respond to current health and health-care problems, developing and supporting grantmaking strategies to bridge health and health care, and designing programs that impact hard-to-reach and underserved populations.

Ms. Yallowitz envisions a future "in which we direct greater attention to the social determinants of health that affect the health status of far too many individuals and groups in this country. We need to build a culture of health for all to embrace." She came to RWJF from the Jewish Family and Children's Service in Princeton, New Jersey, where she created programs to help older adults live independently. In addition to helping the frail elderly, she also developed a Holocaust survivor program and a Kosher Café. Previously, she worked as a family advocate for older adults, as an assisted living facility recreation director, and as a volunteer at senior centers.

Ms. Yallowitz received an M.S.W. in administration, policy, and planning from Rutgers University and a B.A. from West Virginia University. She is a member of Grantmakers in Aging, the American Society on Aging, and Grantmakers Concerned with Immigrants and Refugees.

Kafui Dzirasa, M.D., Ph.D., is the first African American to complete a Ph.D. in neurobiology at Duke University. His research interests focus on understanding how changes in the brain produce neurological and mental illness. Dr. Kafui obtained an M.D. from the Duke University School of Medicine in 2009 and completed residency training in general psychiatry in 2016. His laboratory was featured on CBS *60 Minutes* in 2011. He has been awarded the International Mental Health Research Organization Rising Star Award and the Sydney Baer Prize for Schizophrenia Research. In 2017, he was recognized as 40 under 40 in Health by the National Minority Quality Forum, and the Engineering Alumni of the Year from the University of Maryland, Baltimore County. He was awarded the Presidential Early Career Award for Scientists and Engineers—the nation's highest award for scientists and engineers in the early stages of their independent research careers—in 2016. In 2019, he was awarded the Alan Leshner Public Engagement Fellowship from the American Association for the Advancement of Science and the Society for Neuroscience Young Investigator award given to the best young brain scientist in the world. Dr. Kafui has served as an associate scientific advisor for the journal *Science Translational Medicine*, and he was a member of the 17-member Next Generation Research Initiative mandated by Congress. He has also served on the Editorial Advisory Board for TEDMED and the Advisory Committee for the National Institutes of Health Director for the BRAIN Initiative. He is the K. Ranga Rama Krishnan Endowed Associate Professor at Duke University with appointments in the Departments of Psychiatry and Behavioral Sciences, Neurobiology, Biomedical Engineering, and Neurosurgery.

Aza Allsop, M.D., Ph.D., is a first-generation American who grew up in Trinidad before living in a number of different states on the East Coast. He studied biology, philosophy, and jazz studies at North Carolina Central University before carrying out social neuroscience research training in the Tye lab at the Massachusetts Institute of Technology (MIT) as part of the Harvard Medical School-MIT M.D. Ph.D. Program. He studies how social information is computed, integrated, and biased in the brain and the resulting impact on cognition and behavior. He also studies the mechanisms by which music and mindfulness modulate social connectedness and stress management. His research is guided by the belief that deconstructing these mechanisms will provide a better understanding of how social groups function and offer critical insights into enhancing the development and function of society at large.

Dr. Allsop is a multi-instrumentalist who is deeply rooted in the experience of music from the African Diaspora. He engaged in formal studies of gospel and jazz music in college and as a Ph.D. student was awarded MIT's Emerson Scholarship to study at Berklee College of Music and has released multiple projects of his original music. He teaches music and mindfulness as tools that help enhance empathy, social justice, health equity, and wellness. To that end, he co-founded Renaissance Entertainment LLC, a company that operates at the intersection of music, science, and community building to promote a culture of wellness. He does research and provides clinical care as a resident in the Department of Psychiatry at Yale University.

Eve J. Higginbotham, S.M., M.D., is the inaugural vice dean for inclusion and diversity of the Perelman School of Medicine at the University of Pennsylvania, a position she assumed on August 1, 2013. She is also a senior fellow at the Leonard Davis Institute for Health Economics and professor of ophthalmology at the University of Pennsylvania. She is the immediate past president of the AΩA Medical Honor Society and currently serves on the National Academy of Medicine Council and the National Research Council Governing Board. Dr. Higginbotham serves as a member of the Finance Committee of the National Academy of Medicine. Notable prior leadership positions in academia include dean of the Morehouse School of Medicine in Atlanta, Georgia, senior vice president for health sciences at Howard University, and professor and chair of the Department of Ophthalmology and Visual Sciences at the University of Maryland in Baltimore, a position she held for 12 years.

A graduate of the Massachusetts Institute of Technology (MIT) with undergraduate and graduate degrees in chemical engineering (Course X, S.B., and S.M.) and Harvard Medical School, she completed her residency in ophthalmology at the LSU Eye Center and fellowship training in the subspecialty of glaucoma at the Massachusetts Eye and Ear Infirmary in Boston. Dr. Higginbotham has served as a member of two federal advisory committees: the Defense Health Board, which is advisory to the Secretary of Defense, and the Special Medical Advisory Committee to the Secretary of Veteran Affairs. She is a member of the Board of Directors of Ascension, serving as a chair of the Quality Committee and a member of the Finance and Audit Committees. She is a member of the Board of the AΩA Medical Honor Society of which she leads the Leadership Development Committee, and associate editor of the *American Journal of Ophthalmology*. She is a vice chair of the National Eye Institute–supported Ocular Hypertension Treatment Study, a randomized clinical trial, recently funded for a 20-year follow-up study of this unique cohort of patients. She is currently a member of the Association for Research in Vision and Ophthalmology, American Academy of Ophthalmology, American Clinical and Climatological Association, National Academy of Medicine (NAM), American Academy of Arts and Sciences, and the newly formed Harvard-MIT Health Sciences and Technology Advisory Board and the Visiting Committee of the Institute of Medical Engineering and Science at MIT.

Dr. Higginbotham is a former member of the Board of Overseers at Harvard University, former member of the MIT Corporation, and a former chair of the Food and Drug Administration Ophthalmic Devices Panel. She is the past president of the following organizations: the Maryland Society of Eye Physicians, the Baltimore City Medical Society, and the Harvard Medical School Alumni Council. She formerly chaired her section of the NAM and is a former member of the NAM membership committee. Dr. Higginbotham, a practicing glaucoma specialist, has authored more than 150 peer-reviewed articles and co-edited four ophthalmology textbooks and continues to remain active in scholarship related to health policy, STEM, and patient care at the University of Pennsylvania.

Ahmara G. Ross, M.D., Ph.D., is an assistant professor of ophthalmology and neurology who completed ophthalmology residency at the University of Pittsburgh, then fellowships in neuro-ophthalmology and glaucoma at the Scheie Eye Institute, University of Pennsylvania. She also has a Ph.D. from Thomas Jefferson University. In addition to caring for patients with both glaucoma and neuro-ophthalmologic disorders, she also performs ocular surgery ranging from cataracts, minimally invasive, and incisional glaucoma surgery.

Dr. Ross diagnoses, treats, and manages optic neuropathies beyond the spectrum of glaucoma, but views this disease as another neuro-degenerative disease in need of sight-changing therapy. Her interests and professional strengths go beyond basic science research with a clinical approach also aimed at addressing socio-economic barriers to the treatment of health care. She joined the faculty in 2017 and is currently funded by a National Institutes of Health K08 Career Development award to investigate the neuroprotective potential of gene therapy directed at retinal ganglion cells and neighboring support cells to treat chronic glaucoma. She is also collaborating on similar research using gene therapy to treat other mouse models of optic neuropathy such as trauma, compression, and inflammation.

Shereka Banton, Ph.D., is a senior regulatory affairs program lead at Johnson & Johnson. In her regulatory affairs role, she works to ensure that her company's medical devices are safe and effective according to the regulations that exist for the products. Prior to working in the medical device industry, Dr. Banton completed her doctoral training in the Wallace H. Coulter Department of Biomedical Engineering at Georgia Tech and Emory University. In addition to her work in biomedical engineering, she studied science policy, interned for the National Science Foundation's Education and Human Resources directorate, and was a presidential fellow for the Center for the Study of the Presidency and Congress, for which she authored a paper related to diversity in STEM. Dr. Banton also co-authored a book chapter with her doctoral advisor Dr. Gilda Barabino on inclusive mentoring as a career advancement strategy for underrepresented minorities in science and engineering. Dr. Banton received both her B.S. degree and Ph.D. in biomedical engineering from Georgia Tech.

Orlando C. Kirton, M.D., M.B.A., is chairman of surgery and surgeon-in-chief at Abington Jefferson Health. Dr. Kirton received his undergraduate degree from Brown University in Providence, Rhode Island, and his medical degree, cum laude, from Harvard Medical School. He served his internship and residency in surgery at the State University of New York and then completed fellowships in surgical critical care and surgery of trauma at Jackson Memorial Hospital, Department of Surgery, and University of Miami School of Medicine in Florida. He joined the faculty at the University of Miami from 1992 to 1999, where he achieved the academic rank of associate professor of surgery and served as the director of the Trauma Intensive Care Unit at Jackson Memorial Hospital and served as the interim director of the Trauma Service. From 1999 to 2016, Dr. Kirton was the Ludwig J. Pyrtek, M.D. Chair in Surgery, chief of the Department of Surgery, chief of the Division of General Surgery, and associate director of the Surgical Intensive Care Unit. He also was chief of trauma at Hartford Hospital from 2012 to 2016. Dr. Kirton's current academic rank is that of professor of surgery and vice chairman of the Department of Surgery of the Sidney Kimmel Medical College at Thomas Jefferson University. Dr. Kirton is a diplomat of the American Board of Surgery with additional qualification in Surgical Critical Care. He is a fellow of the American College of Surgeons, the American College of Critical Care Medicine, and the American College of Chest Physicians, and a member of the Society of University Surgeons and the American Surgical Association. In 2014 the Society of Critical Care medicine bestowed him the Master of Critical Care Medicine distinction. Dr. Kirton has served as president of the Surgical Section of the National Medical Association and the president of the Society of Black Academic Surgeons, and was also past president of the Connecticut Chapter of the American College of Surgeons. He served on the Boards of Directors for the Society of Critical Care Medicine, the Eastern Association for the Surgery of Trauma, the National Medical Association, the Society of Black Academic Surgeons, and the Board of Managers of the American Association for the Surgery of Trauma. Dr. Kirton received a physician executive M.B.A. from the University of Tennessee in 2015. He has published extensively in peer-reviewed, refereed journals as well as authored numerous chapters and textbooks on surgical critical care, trauma, and surgical education.

Stacy Blake-Beard, Ph.D., is a renowned scholar, consultant, speaker, mentor, and coach. Dr. Blake-Beard is visiting faculty at Tuck School of Business at Dartmouth College. She has held a number of leadership roles, serving as the 2016–2019 Deloitte Ellen Gabriel Chair of Women and Leadership at the Simmons College School of Business. Prior to joining Simmons, she was on the faculty at the Harvard University Graduate School of Education. Dr. Blake-Beard holds an M.A. and Ph.D. in organizational psychology from the University of Michigan and a B.S. in psychology from the University of Maryland, College Park. She is the author of two books, *Mentoring Diverse Leaders: Creating Change for People, Processes, and Paradigms* and *Handbook of Research on Promoting Women's Careers*. She has also contributed to *Thriving in the Fight: A Survival Manual for Latinas on the Front Lines of Change*, offering the Foreword. Dr. Blake-Beard's academic research focuses on the challenges and opportunities offered by mentoring relationships, with a focus on how these relationships may be changing as a result of increasing workforce diversity. She is particularly interested in the issues women face as they develop mentoring relationships. She also studies the dynamics of formal mentoring programs in both corporate and educational settings. She also researches and practices in international contexts, drawing from her global experiences. Dr. Blake-Beard has published research on gender, diversity, and mentoring in a wide range of publications, including the *Journal of Career Development, Academy of Management Executive, Psychology of Women Quarterly, Journal of Management Development, Journal of Business Ethics, Human Resource Management Journal,* and *The Diversity Factor.* She is co-editor of a volume focused on women's careers titled *Handbook of Research on Promoting Women's Careers.* She is also the co-editor of a recent volume titled *Mentoring and Diversity in a Global Context.* Dr. Blake-Beard received a 2010–2011 Fulbright Award to support her project "Systems of Sustenance and Support: Exploring the Impact of Mentoring on the Career Experiences of Indian Women," in partnership with the Center for Leadership, Innovation and Change at the Indian School of Business in Hyderabad, India. Her most recent collaboration is with Stanford University's Clayman Institute for Gender Research on their Voice & Influence video series. She has also served as a representative for the Board of Governors for the Academy of Management. Dr. Blake-Beard sits on the advisory boards of a number of organizations, including MentorNet, Teen Voices, the Harvard Project on Tenure and the Harvard Medical School Center for the Study of Diversity in Science, the Boston Museum of Fine Arts, and the Boston Women of Color Group. She has been the recipient of numerous grants and fellowships, including awards from the National Science Foundation, the Ford Foundation, and the Robert Toigo Foundation.

Dr. Blake-Beard has given seminars for and consulted on a wide range of topics, including effectively leveraging diversity, implementing formal mentoring programs, unconscious bias, managing visibility, gender and leadership, effective offering feedback, career action planning, and team building. Her impressive list of clients includes Infosys, Hewlett Packard, Jobs for the Future, the Partnership, IBM, Cisco, the Robert Toigo Foundation, Bank of America, Chase Manhattan Bank, PricewaterhouseCoopers, Swissotel, PepsiCo, Goldman Sachs, Intel, Linkage, AstraZeneca, Eli Lilly, Boston Chamber of Commerce, the Conference Board, Massachusetts General Hospital, Brigham and Women's Hospital, Cambridge Hospital, Boston University, Connecticut College, University of Connecticut, University of Michigan, University of Texas, University of California, Harvard University, Boston Public School District, the Ph.D. Project, the Compact for Faculty Diversity, New Leaders for New Schools, and Working Mother Media.

Laura Morgan Roberts, Ph.D., is an innovative global scholar and consultant on the science of maximizing human potential in diverse organizations and communities. She has published more than 50 research articles, teaching cases, and practitioner-oriented tools for strategically activating best selves through strength-based development, workplace equity, and inclusion. Dr. Morgan Roberts has edited three books—*Race, Work and Leadership; Positive Organizing in a Global Society; Exploring Positive Identities and Organizations;* and *The Alignment Quest Toolkit for Activating Best Selves*—and self-published several poetry collections. She is also a frequent contributor to *Harvard Business Review* and *Academy of Management Review*. Her influential publications and presentations on diversity, authenticity, and leadership development have been recognized by Thinkers50 "On the Radar" (2018) and the Academy of Management. She is the 2020 inaugural recipient of the Academy of Management Organizational Behavior Award for Societal Impact.

Dr. Morgan Roberts currently serves as professor of practice at her alma mater, the University of Virginia, in the Darden School of Business. She earned a B.A. in psychology (highest distinction and Phi Beta Kappa) from the University of Virginia, and an M.A. and Ph.D. in organizational psychology from the University of Michigan. She has served on the faculties of Harvard Business School, Georgetown University McDonough School of Business, and Antioch University's Graduate School of Leadership and Change. She has also taught organizational behavior, psychology, negotiations, group dynamics, diversity, leadership, and career development at the University of Michigan, the Wharton School of Finance, Tuck, Georgia State University, UCLA Anderson, Simmons School of Management, and AVT (Copenhagen). Her family roots are in Gary, Indiana, and Washington, D.C., and she is a member of Alpha Kappa Alpha Sorority, Inc.

Valerae O. Lewis, M.D., is professor and chair of the Department of Orthopaedic Oncology at the University of Texas MD Anderson Cancer Center in Houston. She is also the associate director of the Department of Thoracic/Orthopaedic Center and associate director of the Sarcoma Center. Dr. Lewis is a leader in the field of orthopaedic oncology with particular expertise in limb salvage and pelvic sarcoma surgery in adult and pediatric patients. In 2011, she started the Multidisciplinary Pelvic Sarcoma Program at MD Anderson Cancer Center that not only addresses the clinical needs of this unique group of patients but also works to improve both the clinical and functional outcome of patients with pelvic sarcoma. For the past 10 years, Dr. Lewis has served as director of the Musculoskeletal Oncology Fellowship Program at symposiums throughout the year and is active in the American Academy of Orthopaedic Surgeons, American Orthopaedic Association, the Musculoskeletal Tumor Society, the International Society for Limb Salvage, and the Western Orthopaedic Association.

Nina Ardery is the deputy director of the Harold Amos Faculty Development Program. She has been with the Minority Medical Faculty Development Program and the Harold Amos Faculty Development Program since 1993, and oversees the day-to-day operations of the National Program Office in Indianapolis, Indiana.

Elizabeth Ofili, M.D., M.P.H., F.A.C.C., is professor of medicine in cardiology at the Morehouse School of Medicine (MSM) and chief medical officer of the Morehouse Choice Accountable Care Organization. She is a nationally and internationally recognized clinician scientist with particular focus on cardiovascular disparities and women's health. Dr. Ofili has been continuously funded by the National Institutes of Health (NIH) and industry/foundations since 1994, with a track record in clinical trials that impact health disparities. In 2002, as president of the Association of Black Cardiologists, she led the initiative to implement the landmark African American Heart Failure Trial, whose findings led to a change in practice guidelines for the treatment of heart failure in African Americans. Over the past 17 years, she has led the growth of the clinical research infrastructure and training programs at Morehouse School of Medicine with awards totaling more than $150 million, including serving as the founding director of the U54 Center of Clinical Research Excellence, the Community Physicians Network, the U54 Research Centers in Minority Institutions (RCMI) Center of Excellence for Clinical and Translational Research, and the R25 Clinical Research Education and Career Development Program. Dr. Ofili has mentored more than 30 M.D. and Ph.D. clinical and translational science investigators, many of who remain at MSM. She has mentored more than 25 underrepresented minority STEM undergraduates and high school students through funding from NASA and the Minority Biomedical Research Support Program. She is the senior co-principal investigator of the Atlanta Clinical and Translational Science Institute (ACTSI), a citywide collaborative Clinical and Translational Science Awards Program at Emory University, Morehouse School of Medicine, and Georgia Institute of Technology, along with their partnering health systems and statewide research organizations. Since 2007, ACTSI has engaged more than 673 investigators and 134 postdoctoral and predoctoral trainees in discovery science, training, and community engagement. Dr. Ofili has led successful multi-institutional collaborations through the ACTSI and the RCMI Translational Research Network of 18 Historically Black Colleges and Universities (HBCUs), Hispanic Serving Institutions, and Minority Serving Institutions (MSIs) across the nation, and was lead author of a publication on models of partnerships between HBCUs/MSIs and research-intensive institutions. Dr. Ofili holds a patent for "System and Method for Chronic Illness Care," and is the recipient of more than 20 national and international awards, including the 2003 National Library of Medicine's "Changing the Face of Medicine, the Rise of America's Women," the Daniel Savage Memorial Science Award from the Association of Black Cardiologists, America's Top Doctors by Black Enterprise Magazine, and 100 Most Influential Health Care Leaders by the *Atlanta Business Chronicle*. She has delivered more than 600 scientific presentations and published more than 130 scientific papers in national and international journals. As an Association of American Medical Colleges (AAMC) 2007 Council of Dean fellow, Dr. Ofili led a project on best practices to sustaining the biomedical and physician workforce. She has advised the NIH on diversity in the biomedical research workforce, and currently serves on the Advisory Board of the National Clinical Center (NIH), and on the AAMC Advisory Panel on Research. She is an elected member of the Association of University Cardiologists and is on the Board of Directors of the National Space Biomedical Research Institute.

Olujimi Ajijola, M.D., Ph.D., is an assistant professor in the Departments of Medicine-Cardiology, and Molecular, Cellular, and Integrative Physiology at the University of California, Los Angeles (UCLA). Dr. Ajijola received his B.A. from the University of Virginia, his medical degree from Duke University, and his Ph.D. in molecular, cellular, and integrative physiology from UCLA. His clinical training in internal medicine and cardiovascular diseases/cardiac electrophysiology took place at the Massachusetts General Hospital/Harvard Medical School and at UCLA, respectively. His clinical and research interests revolve around innovative methods to control life-threatening cardiac arrhythmias by modulating the autonomic nervous system. He is also an alumnus of the Howard Hughes Medical Institute's Medical Fellows Program, a recipient of the NIH Director's New Innovator Award (DP2), and a Young Physician Scientist Award from the American Society for Clinical Investigation.

Monica Hall is a program associate at the Robert Wood Johnson Foundation (RWJF), which she joined in November 2018. Her work supports RWJF's focus on developing networks of leaders from every sector who share a vision of what shapes health, and who join together to effect change. She views her work as "supporting tomorrow's leaders and helping to extend their influence and impact in building a Culture of Health." Previously, Ms. Hall was the inaugural fellow in her role as program associate with the Victoria Foundation, which seeks to improve the lives of children and families in Newark, New Jersey. In this role, she focused on youth leadership and development and provided guidance in the areas of education, neighborhood development, and the environment. She also presented more than $2 million in grant awards for 31 nonprofits serving Newark children and families. Her work with advisory boards includes the Aspen Young Leaders Fellowship; Leadership Newark's Junior Fellowship; NJ Jobs for America's Graduates; a National Community Schools Advisory Board; and Newark Thrives!, the out-of-school time collective impact initiative for Newark. She also served as program coordinator for the Abbott Leadership Institute (ALI) Youth Media Symposium at Rutgers University-Newark. During her 3 years with ALI, she coordinated an afterschool and summer program for high school students in Newark, a youth-led college readiness campaign, and a statewide youth listening tour with more than 150 students in seven cities. She also implemented systems for ALI's data collection, program evaluation, and emergency protocols.

Ms. Hall earned her B.A. in Africana studies and criminal justice from Seton Hall University, where she was a scholar in the Martin Luther King, Jr. Leadership Program. She is currently pursuing an M.P.A. in nonprofit management at the Rutgers University–Newark School of Public Affairs and Administration. Ms. Hall is a native of Newark, where she currently resides. She is an active member of Delta Sigma Theta Sorority, Inc., a public service sorority. She founded and is an advisor to Skooled, Inc., a Newark-based afterschool mentoring program, led by local college students, at Central High School.

Lynne M. Holden, M.D., is the co-founder and president of Mentoring in Medicine, Inc. (MIM). MIM is a national health and science youth development nonprofit organization. The mission of MIM is to expose, inspire, educate, and equip students to become biomedical professionals through academic enrichment, leadership development, civic engagement, and mentoring. MIM has reached nearly 52,000 students, parents, and educators from elementary school through medical school and recruited 1,500 health and science volunteers. Dr. Holden provides the overall leadership, creates the organizational strategy, recruits volunteers, facilitates program development, and establishes collaborative partnerships.

Dr. Holden earned her B.S. in zoology from Howard University, graduated from Temple University School of Medicine, and completed her residency in emergency medicine at the Jacobi/Montefiore Emergency Medicine Residency Program. She is a practicing emergency department physician at Montefiore Health System in the Bronx, New York. She is a professor of emergency medicine at the Albert Einstein College of Medicine, where she has served as a co-chair of the Admissions Committee and in various leadership positions in the Emergency Medicine Residency Program, the largest in the country. Dr. Holden serves on several national boards, including the Friends of the National Library of Medicine and the City University of New York School of Medicine. She is active in the National Medical Association on the local, regional, and national levels.

MIM has earned 60 press features, including in *JET*, *Essence*, and *The New York Times* and on CNN and FOX News. Dr. Holden has published extensively and received numerous awards for her work, including the Maybelline NY-Essence Empowerment through Education Award (2007), Society of Academic Emergency Visionary Educator Award (2008), Robert Wood Johnson Foundation Community Health Leader (2009), *The Washington Post* Root 100 Leader (2010), Lifetime TV Remarkable Woman (2010), American Medical Association Inspirational Physician (2016), and United Hospital Fund Distinguished Community Service Award (2019).